Befriending THE Wolf

Befriending
THE
Wolf

*The Guide to Living and
Thriving with Lupus*

Milly Diericx

New York

Befriending THE Wolf

The Guide to Living and Thriving with Lupus

Published in New York, New York, by Morgan James Publishing. Morgan James and The Entrepreneurial Publisher are trademarks of Morgan James, LLC. www.MorganJamesPublishing.com

The Morgan James Speakers Group can bring authors to your live event. For more information or to book an event visit The Morgan James Speakers Group at www.TheMorganJamesSpeakersGroup.com.

Shelfie

A free eBook edition is available with the purchase of this print book.

CLEARLY PRINT YOUR NAME ABOVE IN UPPER CASE

Instructions to claim your free eBook edition:
1. Download the Shelfie app for Android or iOS
2. Write your name in **UPPER CASE** above
3. Use the Shelfie app to submit a photo
4. Download your eBook to any device

ISBN 978-1-63047-874-2 paperback
ISBN 978-1-63047-875-9 eBook
ISBN 978-1-63047-876-6 hardcover
Library of Congress Control Number:
2015918327

Cover Design by:
Chris Treccani
www.3dogdesign.net

Interior Design by:
Bonnie Bushman
bonnie@caboodlegraphics.com

In an effort to support local communities and raise awareness and funds, Morgan James Publishing donates a percentage of all book sales for the life of each book to Habitat for Humanity Peninsula and Greater Williamsburg

Get involved today, visit
www.MorganJamesBuilds.com

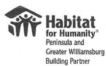

Peninsula and
Greater Williamsburg
Building Partner

To my family

The one I was given
The one I brought forth
The one I choose with whom I share my life

Table of Contents

Foreword   ix

Introduction   xiii

The Essential Triad   xiv

What Color Is Your Reality?   xvi

Chapter 1   Solving the Mystery   1

My Story   2

Ignorance Is Bliss   6

"I Think She Has Lupus"   13

Turning Point   20

From Last Rites to Recovery   25

Chapter 2   Finding Answers   28

Discovering Myself through Research   29

Changing Paradigms   30

Defining Lupus in My Own Terms   32

Chapter 3   Choosing the Path to Wellness   35

Identify Your Triggers   36

Life Situations and Physical Exertion   37

	Hormonal Fluctuations	45
	Spiritual Wellness	46
Chapter 4	**Taking Control of Your Health**	**53**
	Exercise Your Ability to Choose	54
	Cultivate Stick-to-itiveness	55
	Keep Your Thought Patterns Positive	55
	Set Small Goals	56
	Stop the Emotional Roller Coaster	57
	What is the worst that can happen?	60
	What can I do about it at this time?	61
	What am I really afraid of?	61
Chapter 5	**Vanquishing Negative Emotions**	**66**
	The Physical and Mental Level of Emotions	67
	Identify Negative Emotions	72
	Change the Beliefs That Feed Your Thoughts	76
	Choose Happiness	87
	Liberate Negative Emotions	88
	Orient your body and your life.	89
Chapter 6	**Staying Well, Living Life**	**91**
	Tips for Minimizing Physical Symptoms	92
	Alternative Treatments, Therapies, and Diets	102
	Balancing Your Body's Chakras	118
Chapter 7	**Adieu and Godspeed**	**134**
	Resources	**137**
	Bibliography	137
	Web pages (recommended)	138
	Acknowledgements	**141**
	About the Author	**143**

Foreword

By Chloe Faith Wordsworth,
Founder of the Resonance Repatterning® system

Twenty-five years ago I was teaching a Resonance Repatterning seminar in the UK. One of the participants was a Colonel in the British army. He told me something interesting that I have integrated into my work and life, and Milly – consciously or unconsciously – has integrated into her life to help her manage the painful and debilitating disease of Lupus.

The Colonel used to work with survivors of prisoner of war camps. He observed that those who survive the stress of this trauma were not necessarily the healthiest or the strongest. But they all seemed to have three characteristics in common:

- A positive attitude
- A positive response
- A positive concept of time

If we look at these three characteristics more deeply, it will help us appreciate Milly's story and her amazing capacity to transcend the pain and paralysis of her incurable disease.

A positive attitude makes it possible for us to accept that every circumstance, no matter how challenging, always has a higher purpose. Knowing this, and resonating with it, impacts our body chemistry, our immune response and even our capacity to survive life and death situations.

A positive response makes it possible for us to experience that even though we may have no control over life events and painful circumstances, we do control how we respond to these circumstances. How we respond is the difference between a damaging stress reaction and a life-giving relaxed response. When we choose how we respond, we become receptive to inner and outer resources that help us through the most difficult of situations.

A positive concept of time makes it possible for us to resonate with every experience as having a beginning, middle and end. One of the worst things about pain and illness is the feeling that we'll have to live with it for the rest of our life. Maintaining a positive concept of time – that "this too shall pass" – boosts our immune system and helps us access inner resources of hope and resilience. Accessing any positive resource opens a window to feelings of optimism, which in turn leads to empowered action in the face of our challenge.

Milly describes how her "Lupus immune system" is confused, randomly attacking organs, muscles and tissues. Her immune system had lost its natural capacity to recognize a foreign invader. Under any kind of stress, not knowing the invader, her immune system turns on her body's own tissues and destroys them.

Combining both medical and alternative support, Milly shares how she learned to handle the wolf of Lupus, and transform her life from total debilitation to fulfillment.

For myself, after 45 years in the alternative health field, I am convinced that the body-mind has the capacity to heal itself of any disease. But it takes work and commitment: we need to keep our mind open to discover any alternative possibility that might help; we need to be willing to experiment, safely, using our illness as a laboratory to know what supports our healing and what doesn't. We need to go into action to regain and maintain our health over the long haul – for the rest of our life.

Drugs may help in the short run. They may save our life, as they did with Milly. But drugs don't cure. Re-aligning body, emotions, mind and spirit with Nature always leads to self-healing on one level or another.

Milly's book tells her extraordinary journey – from ice baths to bring her temperature down to the Lupus attack that left her paralyzed, in excruciating pain and what the family doctor thought would soon be her death. On her journey back to life, Milly discovered everything that helped her manage this so-called incurable disease – using both medical support to save her life and alternative methods for her long-term healing.

Milly's book, besides being an amazing story, will help anyone with a serious illness and all those learning to live with the "wolf" of their suffering, offering as it does different perspectives, discoveries, possibilities and hope.

If we are committed to our healing, our mind will be open, our intuition will be honed and we will be guided towards our next self-healing step – perhaps a suggestion from a friend, something on the internet or a book will be the tipping point. For instance, David Perlmutter, MD has written a fascinating book – Brain Maker – on the power of gut microbes to heal and their impact on the immune system. He describes how even an incurable disease such as MS went into total remission after treatment. This is only one example of how, as new information pours in, what was deemed incurable in the past is now being cured.

There is always hope! And this is what Milly's book brings.

Introduction

Autoimmune diseases are very prevalent in modern society, and one of the most insidious of these is lupus. The Lupus Foundation of America has estimated that 1.5 million Americans and five million people worldwide suffer from lupus. Of these, 90 percent are women. Other statistics reveal that 65 percent of lupus sufferers live with chronic pain, 61 percent have suffered constraining lifestyle changes, and 50 percent have emotional problems relating to the disease.

According to the American Autoimmune Related Diseases Association (www.AARDA.org), about 50 million Americans suffer some form of autoimmune disease. Although a lot of medical research has gone into these ailments, most of them are still a mystery. Doctors can only deal with the symptoms people suffer, doing their best to increase the life expectancy of their patients and reduce the severity of their complaints.

However, unable to detect a cause, they are not able to cure these often life-threatening illnesses, and the medications prescribed to lessen the symptoms can have uncomfortable, even severe, side effects.

This book was created to help sufferers from these types of chronic illnesses find relief from pain and live fulfilling lives with as few constraints and medications as possible.

If this seems impossible, be encouraged: I have done it myself, and I will share with you how I came to live a normal, complete, and purposeful life. I will tell you what has worked for me to make life a happy, mostly symptom-free occurrence.

My research and experience is about systemic lupus erythematosus, since that is my ailment, but the practices and tips I share in this book will work for all autoimmune disorders.

The Essential Triad

The secret to well-being is balance. We have to maintain balance between our physical body, our mental-emotional state, and our spiritual understanding. This is the essential triad of a healthy, fulfilling life. The body is the final recipient and manifestation of imbalance, and bodies with autoimmune disorders take a very fast, obvious, no-nonsense approach to letting us know we have become unbalanced, medically labeled a flare-up of the condition. Every flare-up is dangerous, because every time the immune system goes into hyperactivity, it is a potentially life-threatening situation.

The secret is to keep the flare-ups to a minimum, and if they do come, to catch them at the very start. Action at the onset inhibits the full-fledged attack and minimizes the discomfort and risk. This is the goal. To attain this goal, we have to know ourselves incredibly well. We have to be familiar with our bodies and their red-flag warnings, and we have to keep our mental-emotional health in balance.

Emotional factors are well known and documented triggers for autoimmune flare-ups, and whereas we cannot control our reactive emotions, we can certainly learn to channel them into non-harmful and even productive outcomes. Emotions are reactions to stimuli. Sometimes the stimuli come from the outside (a threat, an accident, something someone says or does). Sometimes the stimuli come from inside, usually through a negative thought pattern such as worry or stress, or even a reaction to an interpretation of reality.

The emotion can be a positive one, such as happiness, tenderness, or excitement, or a negative one, such as anger, sadness, or frustration. These are labeled positive and negative in relation to whether they make us feel comfortable or uncomfortable. In reality, there are no good or bad emotions; they all have a reason for being. They all are important and are part of our biological kit.

Inhibiting any emotion has consequences: The energy of that emotion doesn't disappear. It remains in the body if the emotion is not expressed or until something is done to channel that energy. Being aware of what we are feeling, whether we like or dislike a certain situation, person, or activity, is extremely important. First, we have to be able to *recognize* our feelings in our bodies. Then, we have to know how each one is *felt*, and in which part of the body. Then, we have to *name* it to ourselves, *accept* that we are feeling this emotion, and finally *do* something about it.

What Color Is Your Reality?

Thoughts are the stories our mind tells us continually about what is happening in the outside reality. Our thought processes are our mind's way of making sense of the world. The mind absorbs information about reality through the senses and then runs this data through its memory bank looking for similarities. When it finds something similar, it triggers the emotional response that was triggered in the past, usually the one that worked in a similar situation.

Our thoughts are not the reality of the situation, but our own personal coloring of what is going on, full of our history and interpretations. Being able to see this mechanism makes reacting to certain situations more of a real experience and less of our own historical approach to life. Knowing ourselves—particularly our automatic responses to stimuli and the emotions created by our thought processes—is an invaluable tool for maintaining mental and emotional balance.

The spiritual aspect of the triad is the frame in which we structure our story, where we find meaning and purpose for our life and its circumstances. Finding meaning is the most effective way to cross the rough patches of life with the courage to go on.

Viktor Frankl in his book *Man's Search for Meaning* narrates how, if you find a purpose to your existence, you find the courage to survive in the direst of circumstances. Dr. Frankl was arrested by the Nazis in 1942, separated from his wife, and sent to a concentration camp. There he observed that people who found meaning in their lives tended to survive, whereas those who lost hope died soon thereafter.

Dr. Frankl set his purpose in surviving to see his wife again. He told himself that even if she were already dead, he would not lose hope, but would continue living. He survived the camp, and although his wife had indeed died, he went on to create a therapy from his findings. Through Logotherapy, he has helped many people find their own meaning and purpose.

Just as Dr. Frankl found his purpose for living, you will have to find yours. I call this a spiritual path. What gives your life meaning and fills you with joy independently of anyone else is probably the purpose of your life. I do not adhere to any particular religion, but I find that people with faith have meaning in their lives. Many ways and paths give meaning to existence, and you have to find yours. Having a good sense of humor and being compassionate and understanding of yourself are necessary for building your spiritual frame of reference.

I will first go into my own story to give hope to those who have it rough and are convinced that there is no way out of the helplessness and depression. There is, and I will show you what worked for me. I will summarize the alternative therapies and treatments I tried and explain whether they worked.

Lastly, I will share some easy, do-it-yourself ways to maintain balance in your body, your mind and emotions, and in your spirit (your life purpose and meaning). This will help to make the good times last longer and the rough patches be much shorter and less painful, until you discover your own perfect balance to keep yourself healthy and happy. This is your body, and it is the way it is. This is your time. Your life is the only one you have. Would you rather spend it being miserable, or being the best you can be right now, right here with what you have?

Let's discover how to make that happen right away!

CHAPTER 1

Solving the Mystery

M y path to inner knowledge has not been a straight one. It has been fraught with turns, pitfalls, obstacles, and surprises, as any journey is. Instead of letting lupus destroy me, I decided to take it as my particular road to finding my higher self, my true self, and my inner balance. I have chosen a difficult path in having lupus, granted, but it is nonetheless a walkable one.

So my path begins not with the diagnosis of lupus when I was thirty one but when I decided to give this condition meaning from a spiritual standpoint. This meaning brought with it a greater love for myself, and I stopped seeing it as a punishment, for this condition brings with it a great gift: self-awareness. If you have ever been a spiritual seeker as I have, you have heard this a million times: self-awareness is the key to spirituality, which is why meditation, contemplation, and prayer are so valuable.

There came a time when I realized that I had my own inbuilt "know-myself" mechanism. I did not need to go to an ashram in India (although I would love to) to find my path, and my guide is my own body. It tells me every time in no uncertain terms when I am doing something that is wrong for me, and it also lets me know how good it feels when I am doing something right.

Yes, I believe that my soul chose lupus to learn this most valuable lesson of giving my being the gift of awareness, compassion, and empathy. This is the meaning and purpose I have found through lupus.

Everyone has to find his or her own higher lesson to be learned; it may be the same as mine, and it may be different. Looking at lupus in this light has given it meaning and purpose in my life.

Although I can't remember exactly the timing, I will attempt to make a chronicle of the events that led me to this befriending of lupus as my guide. It may not be an accurate historical account because I have a terrible memory for facts, as many of us with this condition do. I retain in my mind only what that experience brought me. This is my story as I recall it today.

My Story

My parents were coping with a lot of drama when I made my appearance in the world, in Mexico City, during the summer of 1969. I have an older brother and a complicated but very loving and protecting nuclear family that was wrought by tragedy, especially at the time of my birth, which is why our nanny played such an important role in my childhood.

One of my earliest recollections is swaying back and forth on a rocking chair cradled in loving arms. My nanny was giving me my bottle, sweet chamomile tea, to calm me down and put me to sleep. She was a lovely person with no children of her own, so she loved my brother and me and as a mother would. I remember her infinite patience and care of us. Every night she rocked me to sleep with my bottle of tea. I must have been around three. In this particular memory, I am wearing pale yellow-footed pajamas with a pink bunny rabbit embroidered on the top, and I am comfortable and warm. I can still smell the face cream she used and feel the motion of the rocking chair. I remember grabbing her hand and putting it on my knee, asking her to rub it. She would laugh and ask me if I had rheums, to which I would solemnly nod and move her hand in a circular motion on my knee. The right knee was always more painful, especially at night, after running around all day.

I also remember my skin being very sensitive to the sun. I was a child in the pre-sunblock era, so when we went to the beach, I got blistering sunburns really fast. My nanny, an expert in home remedies, always rubbed vinegar and egg white on my raw skin, making it hurt less. I was the only child in the pool area wearing a T-shirt and a hat to protect my skin from the sun as much as possible.

My skin was always a problem. As a baby, I developed mysterious blotches, had really bad diaper rash, and periodically, I was covered head to toe in little red eruptions. Oatmeal baths and cornstarch to powder me afterwards were the home remedies used on me since no dermatologist could accurately diagnose me. The symptoms were similar to those caused by herpes, nervous eczema, allergies, heat rash, measles, and every other virus that manifests with fever and rash. I was even told once by the local dermatologist that my bed bugs were angry and didn't recognize me anymore. This was by far the more accurate diagnosis; he only got the culprit wrong!

These symptoms were life-long afflictions for which every diagnosis, available medicine, treatment, and home remedy was applied. There were also the mysterious fevers. The first time I got one, I was a year old. My grandfather had died recently, the last in a series of tragedies in the family within a short period. We had moved to Cuernavaca, a small town about two hours' drive from Mexico City. Suddenly my temperature rose uncontrollably to 42 degrees Celsius (107.6°F), dangerously high because it can damage the brain.

The pediatrician based in Mexico City came to see me and was very alarmed at my condition. He gave me every medicine he could think of to no avail, so I was put into a tub with ice water to lower my temperature. When I was taken out, my temperature rose again, so I was submerged in the ice water on and off for four or five days. (No one can tell me for certain.)

The pediatrician made the trip from the city to my home every day to see how I was faring. I could not be taken out of the ice long enough to be taken to his office in Mexico City. He didn't have a lot of hope for me, and my mother probably didn't either, but she would not give up and kept to the ice water regimen until the fever abated as suddenly as it had come. The doctor said it must be a rare virus that gave no other symptoms. I suffered many of those mysterious fevers throughout my life, in varying degrees of heat and duration, making an accurate diagnosis incredibly difficult.

I slept a lot when I was a child, more than the rest of my friends, especially as a teenager. I would get twelve to fourteen hours of sleep every day, and if I didn't, I could not make heads or tails of anything. I do remember being tired many times, apparently more tired than everyone else, even when we had done the same activities, but I thought nothing of it. When I started going out at night, I needed almost the entire next day to recuperate. On my high school graduation trip, when my friends and I went out every night for a week, I lost consciousness for the first time because of physical exhaustion.

High school graduation for my fun group of friends was party time! We organized a trip to Acapulco, no parents allowed, to live it up and say a proper good-bye to our school days; after all, we were adults now! In Mexico, you are an adult in every respect at eighteen. You can go out anywhere, drink, do whatever you want, and supposedly, you are responsible for yourself. I was all dressed up and ready to go dancing again. We had been partying nonstop the entire week, out every night, in the sun all day, getting very little sleep; since my friends were not ready yet to go out, I lay down, just for a little while, feeling quite drained and exhausted but unwilling to stay behind and miss all the fun. I closed my eyes and woke up the afternoon of the next day, thinking I had just blinked and opened my eyes. I was still dressed to go out and very surprised to see my mother there with a doctor, terrified. My friends had been unable to wake me, and I had run a high fever, so they had panicked and called my mother to come get me. I had tests, but not knowing what to look for, nothing out of the ordinary was found except for a high count of white blood cells. They thought I'd had another one of my unknown viruses caused, justifiably, by extreme physical exertion, and life went on.

Ignorance Is Bliss

Fortunately, and I am truly thankful for this, I was not diagnosed until much later. My life would have been very different if I had been. My parents are very loving people who tend toward overprotection. Had they known that I had a condition called lupus, with its odd variety of symptoms, I probably would have grown up in a darkened room, safely ensconced in a disinfected bubble. My life, however, went on normally. I even got to do many things other kids never do, like traveling extensively, for which I am blessed and so grateful that it brings tears to my eyes.

In my case, ignorance was bliss, and my life was a very active and happy one except when I had symptom flare-ups, but when they passed, they were catalogued as special occurrences and forgotten.

My father is hyper-reactive and has always suffered from skin problems, so my condition was thought to be hereditary. (Autoimmune diseases do run in families, so this assumption was right.) He also has knee problems, and has had surgery on both knees, so my joint problems were also thought to be his legacy. The fact that my knees didn't hurt in the same place as his was never taken into consideration, even though the same doctor performed surgery on my knee. When it continued to hurt, we just thought the surgery had not been successful.

At this point, I was still an overprotected, spoiled princess with absolutely no interest in self-awareness. I dated, went out with friends, got up to no good, rebelled—I was the classic teenager.

I went to pre-university at Oxford, where I wanted to study literature and become a writer. I fell in love passionately and was brought back to Mexico to avoid an untimely marriage and got my heart broken in the process. This distancing from my love brought me down into a severe depressive episode, during which I had no energy to get out of bed. My parents thought it was just teenage love and saw no reason to take me to a doctor for broken heart blues. This was my first major bout with depression. Life had absolutely no meaning anymore.

After months of listlessness and lying in bed, I moved to Mexico City to attend college, which got my spirits back to a semblance of normality. I have always loved to study. I fell in love again, this time with a boy from Mexico, my brother's best friend at the time and my husband to this day. I married at the reasonable age of twenty five, moved to New York, and had a wonderful time in the city. I worked as a volunteer at the National Resource Defense Council and with homeless children in Harlem. I got my taste for helping others during this time in my life.

In New York, my skin got worse, and with my hands frequently immersed in soapy dishwater, my skin literally fell apart. We assumed it was an allergy to the soap because I had never done dishes before this. (I was a princess, remember?) I slathered copious amounts of Vaseline on my hands then put on cotton gloves with rubber gloves over those just to take a bath and to clean our tiny, lovely apartment.

This was the first time doctors thought my symptoms might have something to do with the immune system. They gave me cortisone ointments, which, of course, made it better. I also tried the first alternative method in a long line of many. I found a doctor who took one week's worth of urine and made auto-vaccines from it. I injected a daily dose for a month. It seemed to help a little—either that or the cortisone ointments did the trick, or the attack passed, but eventually it also went away.

After two and a half years of a blissful New York life, in which I was spared doing dishes, we came back to Mexico. We wanted children, and I wanted to be close to my mother for that. I was twenty-seven by then. I got pregnant soon after our arrival. My life was very much on course with my plans up to now. Then I lost the baby. The emotional pain was horrible, and everyone thought the depression that followed was exaggerated but normal, given my sensitive disposition. If I had been so depressed over losing my first love, can you imagine what losing my first child did to me? It was devastating.

I got pregnant again twice and lost both babies, each time falling into deep depression. My doctor was baffled. He could not find any logical explanation for the miscarriages. He even told us that we would be unable to have kids, for I was just not able to keep the fetuses. This was a terrible blow, for we had always wanted children, but all the pain of the miscarriages had made us lose hope. I even told my husband that he should find someone else who could give him a family, since I was obviously unable to do so. He, however, was stoic in his commitment and said he would stay with me and we would travel instead. We both love to travel, so we would find professions that would enable us to do that.

We were coming up with these plans when a couple, friends of ours, invited us to a trip to Peru. It was last minute, but we jumped at the chance, tired of the drama about the miscarriages and needing a respite. We visited the legendary Machu Picchu, where I met my first shaman. He was our tourist guide. He gave us all the esoteric details of the ruins and whetted my interest in the mystical world. He took us up to the sacred city at dawn and guided a meditation for us. Without other tourists around, and in the quiet of the majestic Andes Mountains, you can definitely feel the power of the place. It was no wonder to me that the ancient Inca had founded their sacred city on this peak, even if construction was almost impossible. It is a place of power and magnificence.

Our guide then took us to Cusco, where we visited the ancient city and the fountains of Pachamama, the Incan Earth Mother.

Coincidentally, the three women on the trip all had been unable to have children. The other two were unable to get pregnant, and I had lost three babies thus far. We all splashed in the fountain, drank the water, bathed our husbands, and even took some water for later. We did not necessarily believe in the powers of the fountain, but after all, what could it hurt?

The next day our guide took us to visit a local witch doctor. I remember him clearly. His house was a one-room hut with a wood-burning stove and a mounted condor on the wall. Condors are huge birds, one of the largest flying birds in existence. The witch doctor sat crossed-legged on the floor in full traditional attire, chewing coca leaves. His eyes were red with the smoke in the hut, and he could speak very limited Spanish. He was going to read us the coca leaves.

I must admit we took it as a bit of a joke. When my turn came, I sat in front of him, crossed-legged, on the floor. He took a bowl, gathered a handful of leaves from a little mound before him, put them into the bowl, and handed it to me. I understood partly by spoken word, party by sign language, that I had to do something with it. I do not recall precisely what I did with the bowl or the leaves, but it involved mixing while holding a question in my mind and probably even spitting in the leaves after asking the question out loud.

When I had finished, he signaled me to upturn the bowl in front of him, and the reading began. This was my first official reading by an actual witch doctor. I had dabbled with the tarot as a teen, reading it among friends and making a mockery of the proceedings. This, however, was serious business.

His whole demeanor commanded respect for the reading. So I waited. He spoke for about half an hour, part Spanish, part Inca, mostly unintelligible. What I did get was that my life would take a drastic turn soon, that I would be tested harshly, and if I survived the test, I would have to follow a shamanic path, the path of the healer. He explained that all shamans were tested, and only the worthy survived and became healers. At the time, it sounded ominous but so imprecise it was hardly worth taking notice of. I would understand his words years later.

We came back from Peru exultant, happy in our choice of life: traveling would apparently fill the void of having no children. However, Pachamama had different plans, and from our return in September to December of that year, the three of us on the trip got pregnant. It may be a coincidence, but it made believers of us. So I was pregnant once more, and utterly terrified to lose the baby again. I told no one of this pregnancy, not wanting the worry and pity of the family. Only my husband and I knew about it.

One day, an acquaintance called me to tell me of this wonderful therapy she had just received. To this day, I have no idea why she felt so compelled to call me; we have had only brief contacts through the years. But destiny has a way of giving you what you need. So I called up the therapist and made an appointment. She lived in Cuernavaca, but said she was making a special trip to Mexico City to see three people. She arrived early because the other two people had cancelled and I was her only remaining client that day.

The therapy was called Holographic Repatterning, but its name is now Resonance Repatterning. I had never heard of it, nor did I know how it worked. One of its characteristics is muscle checking (applied kinesiology). When the therapist began checking me, I had no response, which was not good. She tried everything and just could not get me to respond. She was desperate, having come to Mexico City just for me, and being unable to proceed with the session or produce any results.

She asked if there was something that I hadn't told her. I told her I was pregnant, but cautioned her that no one else knew but my husband. So she muscle checked for pregnancy and finally she got a response and proceeded with the session. Pablo was born a healthy baby boy at full term seven months later.

After this beautiful initial session, I decided this was what I wanted to do with my life, so I studied this amazing method while still pregnant. To this day, it is the most effective method I have come across.

One of the things that make it unique is its openness. Chloe Wordsworth, the creator of the method and my dearest teacher, has a curious mind, and she has delved into a myriad healing methods and included them in Resonance Repatterning, making it delightfully inclusive, diverse, and therefore incredibly effective. Every person gets a unique session according to his or her needs, making healing fast and successful.

I became a practitioner of this method and thoroughly enjoyed helping people with it. I had found my calling: I was a healer! The words of the Inca witch doctor resonated somewhere in my mind, and I thought proudly of how I had found myself and my path as a healer through the difficult test of losing the babies. But it would not be so easy—not yet. I got pregnant again and miscarried again; no amount of Repatterning sessions could save him.

I was, however, tranquil in the knowledge that I had one healthy son, so I tried again. My second son, Alejandro, was born in October 2001.

I had a Wonder Woman complex back then. I decided that I would single-handedly do everything—take care of my babies, my home, my practice—and do it all brilliantly. Two months later, I was dying of my first full blown, all-inclusive, virulent lupus attack.

"I Think She Has Lupus"

It began as a fever on December 21. It was the holiday season, and true to my nature, I was busy with the babies, Christmas festivities, parties, shopping, decorating—the usual holiday frenzy. We had yet another party to go to when I began feeling ill. My temperature was rising, and my head and body ached, so I told my husband to go alone. I thought I was coming down with a really nasty flu. By the time he left for the party, I was hallucinating because my temperature was so high, but I didn't say anything to him because I didn't want to spoil his evening. I took some flu medicine and attempted to sleep.

I had a dreadful night. Somewhere in it my husband came home, came into bed, and fell asleep. I never noticed. The next morning he left for work, and I, still thinking it was the flu, got up, packed up my babies, and drove the three of us to Cuernavaca to my parents' house. We planned to spend Christmas and New Year's with them. I don't remember the trip; it was as if I had driven in autopilot mode. I only remember arriving, my mother coming out to greet us, me handing her the children, and practically crawling to my room.

The fever continued all day with no let-up, despite taking aspirins and ibuprofen at my mother's urging. My husband arrived later that day.

The next morning, my skin was all red, as if I had been in the sun for hours, and I had some patches of rash, especially on my face, like a red butterfly on my cheeks. All my soft tissue had ulcers: inside my mouth, my nose, my esophagus, and my stomach and intestines burned as if scalded. I could only eat very bland food. The fever had not abated. We thought it was one of those mysterious viruses I had gotten so frequently as a child, or maybe I had picked up a virus from someone at my son's school.

My husband left for Mexico City on December 23. He was going to pick up his mother to come spend Christmas with us in Cuernavaca, and he had some business in Mexico. He was returning the next day for Christmas lunch. (I was deemed too ill for a formal dinner so we settled for lunch.) Before leaving, very early, he took Alejandro, now two months old, out of his crib and laid him next to me on the bed so that I could breastfeed him when he was hungry. Yes, I was still breast-feeding! The doctor said the best protection from any virus for the baby was breast milk, since it has all the mother's antibodies.

When Alejandro woke up and cried for breakfast, I realized I could not move. Every joint in my body was swollen completely, and I could not bend a single one. I lay there, helpless, unable to hold or feed Alejandro. He was bawling with hunger. Every instinct compelled me to move, but I just couldn't do it. I cried right along with him, sobbing in despair and impotence. When finally my mother came up to my room to check on us, we were both a mess: Alejandro had cried himself hoarse, and I was completely exhausted from my efforts to do something for him. She took matters into her own hands, thankfully, and rolled me over to my side, putting the baby to my breast. We both fell asleep. I slept for the rest of the day, just awakened to feed the baby every three hours. My mother slept in the adjoining room to mine to keep vigil through the night, while taking care of Pablo singlehandedly.

Christmas Day came, and with it my husband and his mother. That morning all my muscles were atrophied. My legs and arms were limp, but we had visitors and I felt obligated to go down to lunch. So I was carried downstairs, taking a backward glance long enough to see large clumps of my hair on the pillow, and I was seated on a chair with arms and a high back like a baby's highchair. Everyone tried to be cheerful and nice. I remember only the supreme effort of answering questions through the mental fog and trying to smile.

Finally, the meal was over. I was taken back to bed feeling completely drained and exhausted. My husband took his mother home to Mexico City and stayed with his own family for Christmas dinner. It was obvious my parent's and I could not deal with company at that time.

Everyone was worried now, but all the doctors we knew were on holiday. I refused to be taken to the emergency room, so my mother called a paramedic friend of hers. He said everything sounded very serious, and I needed to see a specialist. He recommended something, but still stubbornly wanting to continue breast-feeding, I refused all medicine. *It will pass eventually; it always does*, I thought.

25th December, Christmas Day. My spinal cord was inflamed and horribly painful, the fever was back to alarming temperatures, my whole body arched in spasms, and I could not deal with the pain anymore. My mother searched frantically for medical help. The only doctor available was a geriatrist whose older patients tend to get sick in winter, so he didn't leave for the holidays. My husband was still in the city, so my parents took me to the doctor's office. He only agreed to see me on Christmas Day because my symptoms were so serious. When he saw me, doubled over in pain, sitting in a wheelchair, unable to move, burning with fever, he was appalled. I sat there listening while my mother recounted the week's events.

Listening to the story, I could not believe it had taken this long to see a doctor. By his face, I could tell that the doctor couldn't believe it either. In my mother's voice, I could hear despair, guilt, helplessness. He could hear it too because he didn't say anything to the fact that we had waited this long. He just uttered the ominous pronouncement, "I think she has lupus, an incurable disease, and by your account, she has an incredibly virulent attack. She has only a couple of days to live." *Merry Christmas!* was my only coherent thought, or the only one I remember. Silence reigned. Everyone was in shock. It took a few minutes to sink in. They had to ask the question, of course: "Doctor, is there anything you can do?"

He prescribed prednisone (or cortisone) in massive doses, not with a lot of hope, but he had to do something.

When the initial shock wore off, depression set in and the next weeks were a blur. My parents called my husband with the news and he came back immediately, but I don't really remember him being there, nor do I remember my children being there, or the nurse that was hired the next day to care for me. All I remember is the void, a huge dark void that had become my entire existence.

After a diagnosis of impending death, when you don't die immediately, there follows an endless pilgrimage of doctors, tests of all sorts, second opinions, and general despair and confusion. My family was going berserk, taking me to specialist after specialist, looking for that person who would say something different, something they wanted to hear. They were in a panic.

I was still in shock and so darn sick that I honestly could not give a damn. I felt like a piece of driftwood in an angry sea. Decisions were made for me, I was never consulted, almost ignored, and it was just fine—I had no energy to think, let alone decide. Appointments, doctors, tests all went by in a blur. The inevitable conclusion was the same: I had systemic lupus erythematosus, an incurable and often lethal disease, and the attack was so virulent and aggressive that I would most likely die very soon. Actually, the doctors did not understand how I was alive still. They just flooded my body with huge amounts of cortisone, transplant strength immunosuppressants, quinine (Plaquenil), and kept me quiet. Time would tell.

Finally, we found a doctor with whom I felt a little more comfortable. He wasn't so vocal in his dire predictions, though his diagnosis was the same, but he was a tiny bit more flexible. Also, he spoke directly to me, not to everyone else in the room as if I was already gone. Keeping him as my only doctor instead of a stream of specialists was the only decision I made that was taken into consideration. The rest was bed, a darkened room, the fewer visitors the better, and complete and utter despair.

My body had become my enemy. It was slowly but surely killing me relentlessly. All I could feel was emptiness in my gut, a sense of hopelessness so profound that it was a black hole, swallowing everything else. Even my newborn son did not give me any joy. I could not exit this black hole of self-pity and hopelessness even to care for him. I had no feelings whatsoever. I could not be angry or worried or afraid. I could not love, and I could not care for anyone, not even myself.

This was probably the worst part, witnessing the coming and going of life with a complete lack of emotion, flatlined, as if I was already dead. When the nurse brought Alejandro for a visit I could only think maybe it was better she didn't. I wouldn't be around for long. What was the point?

I would close my eyes and open them again hours later, feeling as if I had just blinked, but in reality I had gone completely, lost consciousness. No one knew if I would wake up or just stay comatose. Each day was the same as the last, each time of day as dull and pointless as the next.

My life had absolutely no purpose. Many times all I wanted was for my treacherous body to get on with it and finish the job. The pain was horrendous. My skin chafed between the sheets. I could not move at all. I was as helpless as a newborn mouse, exposed, vulnerable, weak, in the dark. The massive amounts of cortisone had stopped the attack, and the immunosuppressant medications had my immune system on hold. No further damage was being done to my body. It was trying to fix itself ever so slowly and painfully from the massive weeklong attack during Christmas.

Months went by. My future looked so bleak I could not even contemplate it, my present so meaningless I could not grasp it. I was drowning in depression and self-pity, one moment differentiating itself from the next only because something new hurt or some pain changed in intensity. I knew it was morning because the nurse came in to carry me to the bathroom for my daily ablutions. My room was always kept dark, as one of my no-no's was sunshine. Light was actually painful on my skin, any kind of light, natural and artificial.

My clue to the time of day was the routine of the house. The nurse cleaning my body, feeding me, and giving me copious amounts of pills (not only the hard drugs, but many others to alleviate the side effects of the primary medicines), which took about an hour to swallow, then Pablo arriving from kindergarten, his little voice ringing throughout the apartment. I could hear him running, crashing into furniture on his tricycle, sometimes even falling and hurting himself, crying. All this I heard through the closed door of my bedroom.

He could only come into my room and give me a kiss once he had passed inspection by the nurse and she had declared him symptom free. It is highly dangerous to be with sick people while on immunosuppressant treatments, as any little virus or bacteria can kill you. Thus, my visitors had to be inspected and then let in for a quick visit before being quickly ushered out.

Alejandro, my baby! I could hear when he cried for his bottle, if he was uncomfortable, the nanny singing him to sleep. Quiet tears ran down my face continually when I heard him, but only quiet ones, as I had no energy to really cry.

Alejandro was brought in once a day to see me, fed, bathed, and content. The nurse would put him on my bed so I could watch, paralyzed with weakness, while he wiggled and cooed, wanting to hold him, completely unable to do so. When I cried she took him away immediately, for I had to be kept quiet, emotionless. His baby smell lingered on my bed, making his absence and my disability more poignant.

Those brief daily visits exhausted me so much that I slept the rest of the afternoon. I knew it was night when I heard my husband come home. I could hear him open the gate, speaking loudly (he has always had a strong character, even a bad temper). He would ask about the kids, about the house in general, many times answer a phone call or two and only then, when everything else was taken care of, would he peek in the door.

If my eyes were open, he would come in, try for a cheerful face, tell me the daily report about work and the kids (which he had just heard), and kiss my forehead tenderly. Then he would leave again to have dinner, be with the kids, watch TV, live life.

Life went on around me, never stopping for a second. My babies were growing up without me and they seemed happy and healthy; my husband kept working, giving orders without me; food was prepared, and kids were fed, taken to school, bathed, and played with. My participation was to listen through a closed door to the sounds of life going on without me.

My existence felt futile; everybody could live fine without me. I felt like I was literally stealing air from the world to fill my lungs. It was useless air, and I was a useless user of resources. I would never be able to do anything but exist, weak and inept, a silent witness to the exuberance of life around me.

Turning Point

One day, something changed. I tried to move a finger and was surprised when it responded. I kept trying, and a few days later,

I was able to move a few fingers. Soon (or not—time had taken a completely different quality now), I could adjust my arms on the bed when they got too painful. I was making progress. It was so slow that nobody else noticed, but since I had nothing better to do, I did.

I spent a few minutes focusing on one part of my body, attempting to move it. I became exhausted and had to rest for hours, sometimes even losing consciousness. I kept up my efforts, probably out of boredom more than hope, but I persevered. Finally, I could move my whole arm to the bedside table. My objective: to pick up a glass of water.

The first several attempts I couldn't move it. It seemed to weigh a ton. I do not know how many days passed with me attempting this single objective. Finally, I could hold the glass and bring it to my mouth, splashing my face with the little water it contained because I still could not lift my head to bring my face closer to it. It was a wet success. I kept on trying to move my toes, then my feet. My legs were a huge step; they felt so big and heavy! But finally I could shift around in bed and get on my side.

One morning, I was feeling extra adventurous, so I turned to my side and let my legs drop to the floor. It felt like a thousand pins and needles had pierced the soles of my feet, and I cried out in pain.

I had to wait for my nurse to come in so she could lift my legs back into bed. That little effort cost me not seeing my children that day; I was so exhausted, I was out like a light.

I regained consciousness somewhere in the wee hours of the night. I knew it was very late because of the quiet. Night was rarely this quiet, always some traffic outside, some creaking of wooden floors, the elevator going up and down. But this night was completely quiet. I wondered if I had finally died. I wondered if my efforts to move had finally been too much for my ravaged body. I wondered all this in complete inner peace. I had come to accept my own death. Vaguely I thought about my children, and wondered if they would notice I was gone from their lives, if they would ever wonder how it could have been. I knew they were fine; I had watched them go on without me, so it was a wonder without concern, just nostalgia for the life not lived, for the caresses not given or received, for the time not spent in their company . . . maybe a minute of regret for my unfortunate demise . . . nothing more. I closed my eyes again, peaceful, even relieved.

But fate had a different plan. I had not died. Next morning, routine came again, the bathroom, the medicines, all of it. At first I was completely desperate. Why was I still alive, still in pain, still in this useless body, when it had all been so peaceful? I was angry now, angry at the injustice of my life, angry at God, angry at my body that would not just pack it up and go already!

When I realized this anger, I knew something had changed within me. I had been unable to feel for what seemed like forever. Anger was good; it gave me strength.

I turned on my side and dropped my legs again, expecting the pins and needles, bracing against the oncoming pain, staying with it. I pushed myself to the edge of the bed. My body felt made of lead, so heavy and uncooperative, but I used the strength that anger gave me and leaned forward, pushed off with my arms, and stood. Only for a moment, mind you, for my legs would not hold me, and I fell back on the bed. I was exhausted but triumphant. I did sleep the rest of the day, but I didn't lose consciousness again.

The next day I tried again, and the next. One of these trials culminated in a step forward. Eventually the time came when I could walk from the bed to the bathroom and back, drained.

One day I asked the nurse to let me bathe on my own, sitting on a stool inside the shower and putting my head down between my knees to shampoo my hair because I could not lift my arms up to my head. When I did touch my own head, I noticed my hair was almost gone. It was coming out in chunks, the shower filled with brown masses of it.

I started to cry, feeling horrible and helpless. I could imagine myself looking like a zombie from a cheap movie, hair in chunks, skin falling off, stumbling around. What could be the purpose of living like this? No answer came, just the sound of my sobs and the running water. I didn't notice or care at the time, but I was actually sobbing. Emotions were coming back.

The nurse came to my rescue again and finished bathing me. I didn't even notice her handling my body and taking it back to bed. My body had become completely alien to me in the past several months, a separate entity that persevered in surviving, that could be moved around and manipulated without me noticing except when it hurt. Pain got my attention like nothing else could.

But not this day—today, my attention was completely taken over by a single thought: *I would rather die than live like this.*

This thought became a decision. I had made my first real choice since the illness. Everyone around me thought I had chosen death because I refused to continue with the interminable list of things I wasn't supposed to do. I even threw most of the drugs away, all the ones that were not essential.

Without realizing it consciously at the time, I had made the opposite choice. By refusing to live in pain, despair, and fear, I had chosen life, real life.

The next few days were filled with arguments. My family could not understand my actions. They begged me to keep to the medical regimen and to adhere to their list of dos and don'ts, which was so extensive that it even included never having a strong emotion again. I kid you not! Basically they had condemned me to a life in a darkened room, emotionless and alone, dead, buried alive. I refused to live this kind of life. It was an existence so governed by fear that it was completely paralyzing, meaningless, numbing, and utterly useless. My family didn't understand my resistance because they were terrified. Hospitalizing me to make me follow doctors' orders was discussed and mercifully not enforced. I would have been unable to stop them if they had decided to do so. They finally, albeit very reluctantly, agreed to respect my decision.

As this was unchartered territory, the doctor could not support me, not with me refusing most medications. So I set forth to seek health in other venues.

I reached out to a Reiki healer, who came every day and gave me a full Reiki session, after which I had enough energy to get up, shower, change and come back to bed. Eventually, I was able to play a little with Pablo, who was three years old now.

I kept to my efforts of doing a little more for myself every day, even if it hurt. Sometimes I got carried away and overdid it, and ended up exhausted for days, unable to move again. But I continued trying, getting to know this alien entity I was trapped in: my own body.

I tried other methods too. By this point, I had attempted homeopathy, acupuncture, Bach's Flowers and SCIO (Scientific Consciousness Interface Operations system). I will go into their description and efficacy later in the book.

From Last Rites to Recovery

My parents were very present during my recovery, being a comforting presence for me and my children. We used to visit Cuernavaca very often because Pablo, a very active little boy, could run around the garden and swim in the pool. He needed a lot of exercise and attention, and Grandma was very eager to give it to him and help me out. My husband did his best, working to pay the twenty-four-hour round of nurses for me and for baby Alejandro, attending to the kids and trying to be there for me. There wasn't much he could do for me personally, but all he could do, he did. I am truly thankful for this support system that kept things up and running, I do believe they were absolutely essential to my recovery, and I send eternal gratitude to them.

February rolled along, and Alejandro was almost four months old and had yet to be christened. My mother-in-law is very religious, and she was getting anxious on this matter. I was waiting to be healthy, but by this juncture, I did not seem to be much better. So we decided to christen him at home with only the priest, the family, and the grandparents in attendance. I was dressed and helped to the living room for the occasion.

The picture of the christening is the only one that I have of that period of my life. My face was so swollen with the prednisone that my cheeks made my eyes close when I smiled. My back had swollen like a tortoise shell, making fitting into clothing a hard and uncomfortable process. I sat throughout the proceedings, still unable to stand. The priest deemed me so sick that after the christening, he gave me the last rites. This frightened me and spurred my will to live.

The realization that lupus is not a curable disease, but a permanent condition that I had to learn to live with, finally settled into my conscious mind. It sounds easy to comprehend this, even obvious and self-evident. For me it was a huge milestone. It meant leaving my Wonder Woman fantasy behind. It meant lowering my self-expectations from perfection to doable. I had the knowledge, but patterns of behavior are not easy to break.

First, I had to change my thinking concerning lupus; I had to see it as a condition and not an illness. I had to accept lupus as a guide, an indicator of my state of well-being, a byproduct of my general hypersensitivity. From this point going forward, every time I became ill, I saw lupus as a new learning opportunity instead of a failure. This was an important change, because now

I was being more compassionate, understanding, and forgiving of myself. Using this knowledge to help others and to help myself gave me a profound mission and purpose for my life.

I realized my concepts and beliefs were all wrong. I had to change them before I could change my behavioral patterns. I found meaning through having a purpose and a dream, always setting new goals, and never giving up on them. I had to find a balance between getting things done and not overdoing it. Balance is the key. To attain inner balance and keep it, you need self-awareness, which is challenging for most of us because our eyes only see out, not in.

I began my quest by reading everything I could get my hands on concerning living with lupus, and by trying alternative therapies and treatments.

CHAPTER 2

Finding Answers

I am curious by nature, so I continued my search. Many discoveries were dead ends, but I tried them all. This long road was incredibly useful, for I got to experience within my body the different effects and degrees of helpfulness of many different therapies. This is how I discovered that homeopathy and acupuncture were great at keeping my body in balance while I am healthy, but they did not do much to alleviate my symptoms during an attack. Reiki and Jin Shin Jyutsu were great at helping me recover from the worst flare-ups because they gave me a boost of energy and eased the pain. We will discuss various alternative therapies and treatments later on in the book.

Discovering Myself through Research

Sometimes it felt like I was plodding slowly through the research, little by little, because my brain was sometimes foggy and I had trouble following a train of thought. Sometimes it got so bad I couldn't even read. Sometimes I could not engage in a simple conversation, losing focus in the first couple of sentences. I could not remember words or form coherent thoughts. My research was therefore sketchy and slow, and I had to read the same thing many times for it to make any sense. I read everything I could get my hands on, from the definition and cause of the illness to every extreme point of view for how to manage it. None of it was very flattering or encouraging.

I understood that medically, lupus is a confusion of the white blood cells, a lack of recognition of the immune system of who you are, what parts of your body are you, and what parts are not. It is incurable and unpredictable, it can attack any organ in your body at any time, without warning. The body has no way of defending itself from it's own immune system, so the attacks to vital organs can be fatal. This is why it is so difficult to diagnose and treat properly, the symptoms are the same as many other diseases, like arthritis, asthma, and all the other autoimmune conditions, all rolled into one and it's unpredictable nature means treatment is tricky.

Psychologically it is catalogued, in milder interpretations, as a severe codependence, as if you are losing yourself; in more accusatory tones, lupus is often described as an attack on yourself because you cannot deal with life and you need someone to take responsibility for you. In psychological terms, the lupus sufferer supposedly has a feeling of being undeserving of love and attention from others, and therefore needs to manipulate them with a life-threatening disease. Lupus is also seen as a misguided form of aggression: you are unable to attack those who really bother you, so you attack yourself. In the more strict circles of energy medicine, lupus is viewed as an "out" of life, almost like suicide, brought on by severe lack of self-love or even profound self-hatred.

All of these definitions do little to bolster your hope and self-esteem! They are all based on the notion that you are somehow provoking the disease, and are therefore guilty of having it. My first difficult challenge was to change these concepts in my own self-view. If I continued to define this illness in such negative terms, I would never be able to exit the infernal circle of depression, guilt, and self-pity brought on by such a mindset. Concepts and definitions, I realized, are just the point of view of different people. Most of them don't have lupus and are defining it only as observers.

Changing Paradigms

Paradigms are changeable, so why not define this condition from the inside, from my point of view. I did not agree that I hated myself and wanted to die. I certainly did not agree that I was continually attacking myself as a manipulation of others, or that I was provoking my illness and was guilty of having it! While sick it is true I could not handle life, when well I was just as functional as anyone else.

What I did find out about myself is that I am more sensitive than most people, especially those who do not have some form of illness, so maybe I do need a little more love and attention than the average person. The best place to get them is from myself though, because others are many times too busy or lack the understanding to give them to me. I do feel sometimes like the world attacks me or rejects me, and I think I have developed a phobic attitude to these feelings! Especially when I'm not well, any harsh words and harsh actions, even on TV, affect me acutely.

Feeling attacked or rejected by the world could explain, on an emotional level, why my immune system sometimes goes on the rampage. It is not trying to hurt me; it is trying to do its job, to defend me, but the "enemy" in the case of feelings is not very clear: they can be triggered by the news, or my children having a fight, my husband speaking aggressively, people rejecting me or treating me differently when they find out I'm sick, anything really. How is my poor very confused immune system, in charge of taking care of me, able to know what is a real attack by external microorganisms and what is a perceived emotional attack by external circumstances? Hard choice, especially at the microscopic level, so when confronted by my feelings of being attacked or rejected, it goes after anything it decides to be the culprit, anything that looks even mildly suspicious, like a knee joint, or a kidney.

My immune system is not trying to kill me; it is just confused as to who the enemy is and this confusion could be aggravated by my own emotional hypersensitivity. In this light, I have seen clearly how my emotional state makes my system go nuts. Hypersensitive equals hyper-reactive. Makes sense, doesn't it? Makes much more sense than the theory that I hate myself and want to attack and destroy me. So definitions are words, mere concepts made by humans to understand and come to terms with reality. So how could I redefine lupus?

Defining Lupus in My Own Terms

Please understand that I am not denying what I have. Denial is dangerous. That was the first thing I tried, for years, looking for shortcuts in the attempt to cure myself, falling for the promises of the cure-all remedies, which don't really cure all.

The only danger I perceived in trying various treatments was that they tempted me to declare myself cured. I did this many times, especially after a successful attempt when I felt really good. I would say, "This time I'm really cured," and go and do something stupid that more often than not would land me with another flare-up of varying degrees of intensity. Do not fall for that trap! Every attack puts your life at risk, and that is something you don't want.

The real gift of alternative therapies was to teach me how to maintain balance in my body, mind/emotions, and spirit. In doing so, I have achieved, if not a cure, a normal life, a life in which I can do what I want to do and feel good on a regular basis. This is not to say I never get symptoms; of course I do, but I know myself well enough to nip them in the bud, getting ahead of the attack, stopping it before it stops me.

Lupus is incurable and potentially deadly, it is true, but you cannot let this knowledge define how you live on a daily basis.

So how do you redefine this horrible life sentence called lupus? I divided the definition into its components and took them one at a time. First I dealt with the lethal aspect, for it is the scariest. What I did was compare it with life. Life itself is an incurable and fatal condition. We are all going to die. My chances of dying of lupus are great, medically speaking, but not greater than anyone else's chance of dying of cancer, a heart condition, diabetes, asthma, slipping in the tub or plain old age. We all have a 100 percent chance of dying, and everyone has to go of something! That takes impending death out of the equation and the definition of living with lupus.

We still have to contend with the definition of lupus as an incurable disease. Let's take disease first. To me a disease is something that attacks the body from outside, like influenza or malaria, caused by microorganisms outside the body. Lupus is a confusion of the immune system, so I redefined it as a condition. Most of the world has a condition to deal with; some people have high blood pressure, others have high cholesterol or elevated sugar levels, allergies, sensitive skin, back pain, hair loss—the list is endless.

Granted, these conditions may seem less severe because their symptoms are less difficult to handle, but some of them are also potentially life threatening, and those who suffer them still manage to lead fulfilling lives. So why should we who have lupus be banned from living? We shouldn't. We just need to take extra care of ourselves to feel well and to do what we want to do. So, even if we cannot entirely rid ourselves of the condition, we can certainly control it and still live very successful, fulfilling lives.

Thus, my definition of lupus changed from an incurable deadly autoimmune disease to *a controllable condition of the immune system*. Sounds better, right? It feels better too. Think about it: you are no longer hating yourself and planning your own inexorable demise by your own inner hand; you simply have a condition you need to attend, like any other.

Now let's deal with how to attend this condition. It is of course unique, and everyone has a particular way of functioning. For this reason, you should try various remedies to see what works best for you. In the next two sections of the book, I will share my experience in terms of recognizing triggers—physical, mental/emotional, and spiritual—and minimizing those through alternative therapies and treatments, as well as lifestyle choices. I hope this will give you encouragement and ideas for practical steps you can take to regain optimal health and inner balance.

CHAPTER 3

Choosing the
Path to Wellness

O n my path to wellness, I discovered that true healing is found in balance and equilibrium, specifically the balance of one's body, mind/emotions, and spirit. Maintaining balance is crucial to maintaining well-being. Although this is true of everyone, it is particularly true of those who have lupus and other autoimmune disorders. When we lose the equilibrium, we lose the well-being. This is our greatest challenge: to know ourselves so well that we can keep the balance.

After realizing this, and the fact that every spiritual system advocates balance and awareness as the key to a higher spiritual way of being, I redefined my definition of lupus:

> *Lupus is a condition of the immune system that is controllable through maintaining balance within the body, the mind-emotion connection, and in spiritual awareness. Therefore, lupus is, to me, a spiritual guidance system that keeps me on the straight and narrow path of balance, well-being, inner knowledge, and self-awareness.*

Wow! That even sounds helpful! When I consider lupus in this light, I am actually thankful to have this condition. It is what I needed to be able to walk the path of balance. When my body acts up, I am reminded that I have fallen off the path, but knowing this, every time I feel sick, the attack is shorter and less acute, and I get myself onto the path of well-being faster. I have not only accepted my condition as a constant companion, but I have befriended it as a sort of guide that keeps me on the path of equilibrium through self-awareness.

Identify Your Triggers

I have discovered that certain triggers cause flare-ups. There are three main categories of triggers: life situations and physical exertion, hormonal fluctuations, and emotional events—especially those times when you are overcome by fear, sadness, or anger. There are, however, counterparts to all of these triggers. Determining your triggers will empower you to find balance and equilibrium within your body and spirit.

Remember, the better you know yourself, the easier is to maintain balance. You can counteract the triggers that signal oncoming lupus attacks if you know what those triggers are.

Having a sense of humor and a good laugh at least once a day is a very invigorating and healing practice because it liberates endorphins, the happiness hormones, which have been proven to reduce stress, alleviate pain, dissipate depression, and make you feel better, no matter the circumstance.

Carla Ulbrich, a fellow lupus warrior, has written a book on the importance of laughter in dealing with this condition. In her book *How Can You NOT Laugh at a Time Like This?*, she writes, "Laughter provides pain relief, lowers blood pressure, boosts the immune system, and even works as exercise."

It is also very important to know what gives you pleasure. What do you really enjoy doing? These can range from activities that involve pleasurable physical exercise, such as walking, running, bicycle riding, carpentry, and gardening to quiet activities such as sewing, crafting, reading, watching television shows, and listening to music. Consider what you enjoy doing that is not so strenuous and that you can do on a daily basis, activities that are restful and relaxing, and you can always rely on them to give you a sense of serenity and calm.

Life Situations and Physical Exertion
- **Prioritize your tasks**
- **Don't overdo it**
- **Get adequate rest**

When I know that I must do something that requires physical exertion, as it often happens in life situations, first I prioritize. I divide my time between what I *have* to do and what I *want* to do, in order of enjoyment, and pace myself through my activities. I always have at least one thing I want to do in my priority list. Doing only chores is depressing. It is important to have one activity to look forward to, even on bad days. This can vary from enjoying a scented bath to calling a friend who always makes me laugh. Always remember that autoimmune conditions take up a lot of energy because our systems are in constant overdrive. For this reason, we have less energy than most healthy people have, and we need to manage it intelligently and efficiently.

I try not to strain my energy or get involved in projects that involve a strenuous effort, such as hiking or mountain climbing. If I have already started a task and need to finish it, I rest later. For example, during a trip I agreed to bike around the city of Berlin with the family and could not turn back until the tour was over. I was tired, but I persevered. I was really enjoying the experience, as was all of my family, and I did not want to ruin the outing for anyone.

After an experience like this, I take it very easy the next day or two, and I try to be especially aware of any symptoms that flare up. The day after our bicycle tour of Berlin, I organized a tour bus of the important historical sites in the city, but I stayed in the bus resting, out of the sun, while my family examined the monuments up close. I also had my cortisone with me in case my symptoms flared up. I only take it when I feel a symptom coming on, and only in tiny doses now. However, you need to know yourself exceedingly well to get away with living medication free and relying solely on your sense of inner balance. If you choose to do so, please consult with your physician or health care provider.

Sleep is very important. I get insomnia often, and I have found that certain natural remedies help, such as melatonin supplements, valerian extract, and sleep enzymes. They work great in combination with relaxation techniques, which I will discuss later in the book.

If these don't work, I go for the over-the-counter sleeping aids. I don't like chemical drugs as a rule, but not sleeping is worse than the potential side effects, so if the natural stuff doesn't work, I do go for the pills. I even keep prescription drugs at hand in case nothing else works, although my doctor knows I try not to take them, and I do so only when I really need them. Make sure you get at least eight hours of sleep every night, more if possible. For me the ideal is nine or ten.

If you feel tired, rest. If you can't rest at that moment, do what is necessary and make sure you rest later. Rest is not a waste of time; it is a necessary factor in keeping yourself healthy. I try to have projects that involve no physical effort at hand to take regular rest times that feel like a treat. For example, I love reading. I have found that giving myself time to get comfortable and immerse myself in a book is an awesome way to rest.

When I am physically drained and my mind is fuzzy, and reading is an effort, I enjoy watching a variety of television series. Knitting, sewing, and drawing are also fulfilling activities if you enjoy them. You can rest your body while darning your socks or replacing missing buttons on shirts. Find something restful you have fun with, and keep it at hand for those times when you feel exhaustion creeping in. This will make rest time treat time or useful time instead of getting-sick time or boring, useless time. The better you feel about yourself, the less difficult it will be to manage your flare-ups and keep your symptoms at a minimum.

The sun is an ever-present trigger, and to top it off, I have become intolerant to sunblock. When the sun is out, I reduce my skin's exposure to sunlight. I always wear long sleeves and a hat, and I always carry sunglasses with me. I have found, however, that photosensitivity is not constant. There are days when sunlight feels like acid on my skin. On those days, I cover up completely, including wearing gloves, and I wrap a light scarf around my neck and lower face. Other days I can go short distances in the sun without protection and have no consequences. It is a matter of trial and error. Like movie vampires, I stick out my hand into sunlight; if it starts smoking, I know it's a photosensitive day and dress accordingly. (My skin doesn't really smoke, of course, but if it feels like it's burning I take the appropriate measures). Always have sunblock with you, a hat, and sunglasses, especially if you live in a sunny climate. Having all your sun protections in your handbag is a necessary step in preparing to go out.

Skin is the largest organ of the body, and it is exposed to all external irritants and factors. Keeping your skin in good condition is a good way to stay healthy. I find that my skin tends to dryness, and when I dry out, the rashes appear or worsen. I moisturize twice a day, preferably with oil, not commercial moisturizers that have chemicals in them. My favorite oil is cold pressed virgin olive oil, but I also use coconut, almond, or grape seed oil. Almond is the thickest of the three. I use it when the air is very dry or I am in heating or air-conditioned environments, which dry me out. Olive oil

I use at home, especially at night, when being greasy is not a problem. During the day, coconut or grape seed are lighter oils that absorb faster and don't make your clothing stick to you and get stained. Always use the edible varieties, not the scented massage oils. If you hate oils, look for moisturizers with all natural ingredients, especially for your face.

Soaps and detergents can cause allergic reactions, and all allergies are reactions of the immune system, and must be avoided. I use natural soaps, detergents with the least chemicals, and I blush to admit, I do not bathe on a daily basis if I don't urgently need to! On the days when I don't take a shower, I use baby wipes to wash the necessary parts and moisturize the rest of my body. On my face, every week I put on a vitamin E capsule directly on my skin. It seems to keep the skin on my face in good condition.

Other problematic body parts are your kidneys. They have to deal with all the medications and the outcomes of the lupus attacks, so they need to be kept as healthy as possible. I take a natural diuretic every day. Black tea and coffee are diuretics, even when decaffeinated. White corn hairs made into an infusion are very good kidney cleansers. Pineapple is a diuretic, and when blended with parsley, it makes a delicious smoothie that helps rid you of surplus water.

The lungs are always at risk of respiratory infections, a major complaint of lupus sufferers. One good trick is to keep your sinuses hydrated. I know it sounds funny, but when your nose and throat are dry, it is easier for viruses to invade. I use a saline solution in spray; you can get it at any drug store. If the air is dry, I put moisturizer or oil inside my nostrils. If it is winter and the heating is on, sleep with a humidifier in your room.

If I have been somewhere where there is a chance of getting the flu, like the kids' school, the supermarket, a movie theater, or anywhere where lots of people congregate, I use colloidal silver to disinfect, preventively. Colloidal silver is a natural antibiotic. You can get it online and in health stores. I put one drop in each nostril and about five down my throat. If you don't have access to colloidal silver, rosemary essential oil, diluted in your moisturizer, also works. If you have access to nothing, wash out your nose with soap and water and do Listerine gargles for your throat.

I did this in an airplane once, where someone aboard was coughing and sneezing. I had packed all my remedies in my luggage so that I could go through security, so I had nothing with me. Every time I went to the bathroom, I washed my hands and the insides of my nostrils, and then I moisturized them. I had a tiny bottle of mouthwash to gargle with, and I escaped contagion. You can even order a drink of vodka and water and gargle with that.

Blood pressure is an issue for those who have lupus because the heart is at risk, and swelling increases the pressure. This is why diuretics are so important. Follow your doctor's orders if you are prescribed blood pressure medication, but you can supplement with herbal combinations that naturally reduce blood pressure. Eating a diet low in sodium helps to maintain healthy blood pressure levels. Canned foods and processed foods tend to have excessive amounts of sodium.

Avoid adding salt to your food; it usually has enough anyway, especially restaurant foods.

Joints, muscle aches, and pains—I have never gotten completely rid of these. I have only managed to reduce them to a tolerable level. To ease pain in your joints, use gentle movements; do not stay in the same position completely immobile too long. At various times of the day, I get up, rotate my ankles and wrists, move my fingers, walk a little, bend down, and stretch my back, rotating the shoulders and neck while I'm bent over.

This keeps my joints from becoming stiff and painful. My major problem areas are knees and shoulders, so for exercise I never use weights or do high impact activities such as running. I stick to walking, yoga, and swimming, which are low impact and move all the joints in the body. For muscle stiffness and pain, a hot bath can do wonders. If you add lavender essential oil to the water, or Epsom salts, it is even better. Regular gentle stretching also keeps your muscles and joints flexible and supple. Homeopathic Arnica is great for inflammation, as is Arnica oil applied topically to swollen joints and bruises.

Even while lying in bed resting, do your joint movements and muscle stretches gently and consciously. In the morning, after many hours of lying down, start by gently rotating your joints and stretching your muscles. If you do this with awareness, you will know whether a part of your body is extra painful or stiff, and then you'll be able to do something about it. Maybe you need to take it easy that day, or you might need to use hot and cold compresses for stiff or swollen joints. For a natural way to soothe stiff muscles, try menthol oil.

Acidity in the body can be a factor in getting ill, and the drugs prescribed for lupus tend to acidify the system. Do anything to balance out the acidity. Mouth and nose ulcers tell you when your system is acid. Having a teaspoon of baking soda and brushing your teeth with it helps to alleviate the pain of mouth ulcers.

Alkaline foods are best for combating the effects of lupus; these include foods with lots of calcium, such as milk and cheese. If you are lactose intolerant, take calcium supplements. Red meat and certain fruits and vegetables are acidic: citrus fruits, pineapple, peppers, and tomatoes. When you are suffering the symptoms of too much acid in your system, avoid these foods. The telltale signs of an acidic body are acid reflux, swollen gums, map tongue (when your tongue has red patches), and ulcers in the soft tissue.

Lymphatic nodes are very important. They are clustered in bunches throughout the body and they are an integral part of the immune system. When a node is swollen or tender, it is a red flag for your immune system, it is telling you that there is an invading microorganism (virus or bacteria) or that you are at the start of a flare-up. Swollen or tender lymph nodes are always cause for concern and you should let your doctor know immediately if you find one.

The most obvious lymphatic tissue collections are the tonsils, but around the armpits, the breasts, the stomach and the inner thighs, we have large concentrations of them. A good way to check them is while you bathe or moisturize. Do it consciously, touching your body with awareness for any little knots or tenderness in a certain area. Doing lymphatic drainage massages is a very good way to keep the lymph nodes clear, and also to find a particularly painful one that should be looked at by a doctor. Exercise naturally drains the nodes and keeps them unclogged. The lymphatic system doesn't have a pump organ, nodes are embedded in muscles, and they get drained when the muscles are active. Movement is therefore vital to keep this very important system functioning properly.

Hormonal Fluctuations
- **Know the timing of your cycle**
- **Pamper yourself a little**
- **Take precautions during pregnancy**

I am very aware of the timing of my menstrual cycles and do not plan anything too demanding for those times. I try to rest and pamper myself, especially during PMS. I usually take the chance to do those things that I want but never give myself time for, like go to the movies, have coffee with friends, get a massage or a facial, or write a book! These activities are positive and make me feel good. They involve no strenuous effort and do not feel like a punishment. I am also extra vigilant at these times for any symptoms that might come up.

Pregnancy is a very risky matter for women with autoimmune disorders. You should consult your physician throughout your pregnancy and stay very aware of your symptoms. Not only is miscarriage a big possibility, but the hormonal changes that occur during pregnancy and after giving birth are huge and potentially a high-risk factor.

Spiritual Wellness

How you choose to attain spiritual wholeness is as personal as your nature. I do not believe that any particular path is superior to another. My motto is this: if it works for you, then it is your path. In my search for well-being in the body, I have tried many spiritual approaches. I have found serenity through meditation. Most modern spirituality is based on this concept.

Meditate to quiet the mind and become aware of the present moment. It is an incredibly useful technique, as quieting the mind and being aware of your body is a necessary step in recognizing the red-flag warnings when your symptoms are beginning. Your body does let you know from an early stage when something is wrong. To listen to it, you must be tranquil and quiet. If you are running around doing things, worrying, over-thinking the situation, chances are you will notice only when your body is in a full blown attack.

I have polished the conscience of my body, of every feeling, perception, and thought, so that I know when one of my triggers is being activated. Only through the quiet mind can you observe yourself. Meditation is a proven technique to do just that. Give yourself time to see how you are doing every day. This is being proactive with the condition and loving yourself. Meditate with no expectations, just awareness of how you are feeling within your body. When something feels wrong, identify it and take action immediately. This is keeping the balance.

There are many kinds of meditations; some are guided with imagery or with sound. All kinds of guided meditations and sound techniques are available online. In this respect, I would advise you to be discriminating in the source of the material; know where it comes from and what intention it has. For example, a good source for sound meditation is the Synchronicity technique created by Master Charles Cannon.

There are also meditations in movement, such as tai chi, qigong, or yoga. You can also take quiet walks in the forest, on the beach, or in a neighborhood park. The best meditation technique is whatever works for you. Try various methods to see what makes you more aware of your body. The objective is to quiet or distract the mind so that you can focus on your body to determine if something is uncomfortable, if you are more tired than usual, what feelings have come up, and how you are coping with them. Keep this goal in mind when looking for meditation techniques. At the end of the book, I include some that I have found useful.

When I talk about spiritual wellness, I do not mean being religious. I do not endorse any set of beliefs. However, a belief system can help you come to terms with your condition, putting it in a realm where it has meaning and purpose along with everything else in your life. Whatever belief system you adhere to, spirituality in the context of lupus is the ability to step back from yourself, from your ego or personality, to watch your body, your thoughts, and your emotions, from the viewpoint of a witness, to gauge their true dimension and do something about them. It also puts you and your condition into a greater perspective, where the essence of being has meaning, has purpose, and is not random.

Spirituality in this context puts you back in the driver's seat. You are the one holding the reins, not your emotional turmoil or mind constructions. From this space you can see that most of your thoughts are nothing but fantasies you construct, and your emotions are the physical reactions to these constructions, and they both have probably very little to do with reality. However, they do affect your physical health. Always remember, your thoughts, emotions, and body are one system, one inseparable entity, and if one is not well, the others will be affected.

Only in the witness stand can you do this, not being part of the action. That is why I always recommend some form of meditation to watch yourself, see your own inner workings, catch yourself feeding your negative emotions with your thought patterns, falling victim to your own storytelling.

Focusing on the here and now, on what is really happening at this moment in my body, is the most useful technique for me. It is similar to Vipassana meditation. It is the simplest, and therefore sometimes the most difficult, of meditations. It implies concentrating, without effort, on the present moment, on how your body feels sitting on the chair, your hands washing the dishes, the temperature of the air on your skin, the quality of the light, your breathing, nothing more. It means just being present, and not daydreaming or storytelling in your mind. Sounds easy and you may even think you are always present. You may be wondering, *where else would I be?*

Allow me to explain. We spend most of our time thinking, being more in the mind than the body. Every time you catch yourself thinking, you have come back to awareness. You are only aware that you left when you come back, as it were, so catching yourself is good; it is a moment of true awareness. Take that moment to do your scan of body and feelings. You really can't force awareness. You can only make the conditions available for it to happen. Meditation is one of the ways to do this.

You can get incredible experiences and revelations through meditation. However, you should meditate without expectation. Wanting something to happen usually inhibits it from happening.

No matter what path of spirituality you take, always remember to check in with your body to see how it is feeling every day.

There is an exercise you can do, called felt sense, to determine what your body needs, what it is up to doing and what it is not up to doing. This "felt sense" as Chloe, who proposes this method calls it, is a very good thermometer for what is good for you and what is not at any given time.

In her book *Quantum Change Made Easy*, Chloe Wordsworth defines felt sense as follows:

> *Your felt sense is not your intuition, neither is it your thought process; it is the physical perception of your emotions through your body; it is an aspect of the kinesthetic sense, just as color and sound are physical perceptions in your body of the sight and auditory senses.*
>
> *Constantly you take in information through vibratory frequencies. Your felt sense is simply the physical consciousness of what you are feeling. It is a physiological*

response that lets you know how you are feeling in any situation. The more you use it, the more present it becomes in your daily awareness, just as seeing and hearing are part of your daily consciousness.

You can use felt sense as a way of taking inventory of how you feel within yourself that day and in any situation. The following is an exercise to help you begin feeling this sense. If you don't get results from this exercise right away, please don't be discouraged; persevere, and your felt sense will become more sensitive and accurate the more you heed it.

Felt Sense exercise (taken from Chloe Wordworth's work):

Stand up and close your eyes. Put your awareness in your body: feel your whole body, your pose, how you are standing, how you are feeling in this moment. Say your name out loud and feel how your body swings gently forward. Now say another name, one of a different gender. Feel how your body tilts gently backward. This response means you are resonating positively (yes) with your name and negatively (no) with the name that is not yours.

Wait for the response to come naturally, even if it takes time. Do not force it or think it. Feel the reaction in the deep, inner core of your being. Practice until you can feel it clearly. Some people tilt backward for yes and forward for no. What is important is that you feel it inside yourself, the natural pendulum-like motion of your body in response to your name.

Once you have this response, you can use it for any "yes" or "no" answer you need for a difficult situation you are facing.

Knowing that your body responds positively or negatively to any given situation makes it much easier to determine whether it is good for you to be in that situation. If you do not get a response, no matter how much you try, don't worry; you might be attuned to your felt sense in other ways, such as undeniable hunches you get about certain situations. Being aware of your felt sense makes life easier.

Felt sense is not to be used to make important decisions in your life, or to diagnose yourself. It doesn't show facts; it just tells you how you feel (positively or negatively) concerning a certain situation. For example, if I ask, *Am I pregnant?* My body might tilt forward. This doesn't necessarily mean that I am pregnant, but it will tell me that I resonate in a positive way to being pregnant. It is however, incredibly useful if I'm trying to get pregnant and tilt backward when I ask that question, because that means my body is reacting negatively to the option of being pregnant, which could inhibit my ability to get pregnant or even my desire to on a subconscious level. In that case, something inside me is either afraid or uncertain, and solving this matter could be very beneficial for me to attain this goal.

Felt sense will always let you know how you feel toward any situation in your life at any moment. That feeling can be different at different times. For example, if I ask whether it's best for me to go to dinner at my parents' house tonight, one day the answer might be no, and another it may be yes.

Your felt sense is a thermometer of your energy at any particular time. Your energy is always changing, and you can do things to change it. YOU are the one who decides, not anyone else, not even your felt sense, YOU, the whole you.

Remember, spirituality is a path, not a goal, because you never stop growing. The most important thing is to get on your path to self-awareness immediately. This aspect of the triad—wholeness and balance between your body, mind-emotions, and spirit—is the only one that will give you true hope, meaning, and purpose. You don't have to become a guru or a saint; just find your purpose and something that gives you meaning. This human existence cannot, should not be a futile experience. It should have some purpose for you; having this condition has taught me so much. This knowledge, this experience has to have a deeper meaning. I choose to give it meaning. So can you; so does yours!

CHAPTER 4

Taking Control
of Your Health

For me, the worst part of this condition is the depression that sometimes gets the better of me and makes me feel impotent to help myself. For a long time, I could not do anything for myself, and that was frustrating. We all need to have hope. Hope is the energy that gets you through bad situations; hope lets you see possibilities. When we are hopeless, nothing seems worthwhile. The main purpose of this book is precisely that: to give hope to everyone who wakes up every day and faces life with an autoimmune condition. It is possible to live better, and to have meaningful and happy lives, not just suffer through them. The first ingredient of hope is the acceptance of choice.

Exercise Your Ability to Choose

In every situation in your life, you always have a choice. I know it is sometimes difficult to believe, especially when you are feeling horrible, but you do. Even if it's only in your outlook on life, you always have a choice.

Try this: when everything looks hopeless and dark, think of how you could see the situation differently. Ask yourself, "What would I like at this time that is different to what I have?" Of course, the obvious answer is health instead of illness, and that is a valuable, albeit general answer. The secret to attaining your goals is making them reachable. Baby steps are more easily taken than huge leaps.

I will mention here the importance of finding a doctor with whom you can communicate openly, who listens to you and works with you, not on you. A good doctor is one who treats you like a person and not an illness, and who helps you help yourself. Another extremely important ingredient is a support system. Usually this role is taken naturally by families, but there are cases where families are not an option. In those cases, look for friends, health care givers, church groups, even someone with the same condition who understands (lupus support groups on line, for example). Not only can they support you emotionally, but they can help keep things going when your symptoms get really bad. Find a good support group to lean on in times of need, and show your gratitude by helping them when they need it.

Cultivate Stick-to-itiveness

Resilience and perseverance are vital qualities that most people with autoimmune conditions develop out of necessity. These qualities are great to rely on as you live day in day out with the changing symptoms and circumstances of lupus. Add to the pot a good measure of humor. Laughter activates the production of endorphins, and it has been proven to relieve stress and even physical pain. Besides, when you think about it, the situations this condition gets us into can be ridiculous!

Changing your point of view to see the funny side of what is happening gets the raining dark cloud away from your head. If you approach life with a sense of humor, you will be much easier to live with than if you are a grouch all the time.

Keep Your Thought Patterns Positive

Thought patterns, the way you think about yourself and your condition, can be healing or destructive. Having a more positive outlook is always a good thing. When you make your definition of lupus as personal and positive as you can, it will definitely change how you think of yourself, and therefore how you think about and experience your life.

This may seem trivial when everything hurts, but it has been proven by science that thought patterns create emotions, and emotions affect the body as well as the general well-being of a person. Change your thoughts, concepts, and definitions to a positive tone. Remember, definitions are made by people, and can be changed by people. You have as much right to define what is happening to you as a researcher has, and many of those researchers have never felt what you feel.

Set Small Goals

Think of something small you would like to have right now instead of feeling bad (if that's the case). This could be making just one symptom better, having a new attitude or feeling, or maybe just having hope and trust that this too will pass. Think of your immediate positive goal and then find one healing technique that interests you and that you can use to accomplish that goal. (I have provided some excellent techniques in Chapter 6.) Choose the technique according to your felt sense. As you do the technique with focused attention, notice any changes in attitude or feeling, and take one small action toward your goal.

For example, suppose your immediate goal is to go to the kitchen to prepare your lunch, because you do have to eat to keep your system balanced and healthy, but you are too exhausted to do it, and it seems like an overwhelming task. Do your chosen healing technique, and when you finish, take the first step toward the kitchen intentionally and with purpose. Odds are you will take the next and the next until you accomplish your goal. After completion, when your lunch is ready, enjoy it thoroughly. It is the prize for your action. Enjoy and congratulate yourself on the best lunch ever! Then set your next small goal.

When things are bad, this is a very good way to prioritize and accomplish the essentials, and to feel good about it in the process! Remember, even if things are bad and your energy level is low, do one activity that is pleasant; pamper yourself at the level you are today. There are many ways to pamper yourself, some of them really simple, like having your favorite chocolate after doing the laundry, or listening to happy music as you sweep the floor. If you have more energy you can take a half hour break to go for a walk, bake cookies, or visit a friend. The size of the action doesn't matter; it is the intention that changes the outlook.

Stop the Emotional Roller Coaster

I get this a lot! I have concluded that lupus is inherently linked to my hypersensitivity, both physical and emotional. I often feel overwhelmed, sad, even under attack by an aggressive and invading world. I am extra empathic, and everything makes me cry. I am definitely hypersensitive to that which goes on around me and inside me. It is therefore extremely important for me to know what triggers my emotional reactions and what to do about them fast. If I let a negative emotion take over, I lose internal balance, and soon I get symptoms.

Emotions are, in a physical sense, chemical reactions to stimuli. Your brain perceives something and reacts by sending the signal for the creation of certain neurotransmitters that initiate a chain reaction of hormones and enzymes that invade your body. This is an emotional reaction. Your brain doesn't do this to antagonize you; it does it to protect you or to help you enjoy, depending on the emotion triggered. All emotions have their reason for being, their usefulness, and their place. Without emotion, we feel dead. We need emotions. They are not the enemy; they are what give our lives color and spice, even the "negative" ones.

However, all the negative strong emotions are potential triggers, so it's incredibly important to identify the cause and do something about it. Repressing emotions is never a good answer; even if they don't make sense, you have to give them the space to be expressed. If the moment you feel them is not a proper moment to express them, take time to recognize them in your daily self-awareness exercise and channel them through appropriate means.

Anger, fear, and sadness are, for me, the most acutely felt and energy draining, but they are easy to identify and have very specific outlets. For example, anger makes you want to scream and hit something. You can try screaming when you are alone (so you don't frighten the family) and/or hitting a pillow; that way you avoid hurting anybody. Sadness makes you cry, so cry, sob and vent all of it out! Fear is a red flag for danger, and danger has to be tended to. It either paralyzes you or makes you want to run or fight. To channel fear you must identify the source, fear of what specifically, what is the danger you are perceiving, and then, if possible, remove the source of danger. An obvious example would be fear of injury in a car crash. To remove the source of danger, avoid driving when tired or feeling really ill. There are others that are more nebulous like fear of death, of failure, or success. These are harder to deal with, since the source is not immediate, but further on we will review ways to deal with them too.

Stress, anxiety, and worry tend to be less easily identifiable, and they linger within you longer. It is more difficult to do anything about these emotions because they usually don't relate to anything specific. They are mental constructions of future catastrophic possibilities. The human mind evolved to construct possible scenarios. It is part of the limbic brain, one of the most primitive parts of our inner computer. Humankind survived the beginning of history thanks to this capability. We became the only animal that developed imagination, the ability to construct mental images of various possibilities, and then to prepare for them. This was essential since we were at a great disadvantage against other species in terms of our physical bodies. We are weaker, softer, slower, and have no inbuilt weapons, like fangs, claws, horns, or armored skin. Our brain grew, and we developed mental skills, imagination, and a sense of time so that we can actually think of and plan the future, as well as remember the past and learn from it. These became our weapons in a world filled with predators and dangers.

Today, however, this ability fills us with stress and anxiety. We tend, as a defense mechanism, to think the worst of any situation, to be prepared. When this situation was a saber-toothed tiger hunting us, this innate skill was immediate and lifesaving. When the scenario is possible world war, it is less useful, for there is nothing we can do about that. The brain function is the same, but we have completely transformed our environment, so threats are not immediate and impending; they are more of a mere mental construction, possibilities that rarely happen. The brain doesn't know there is no tiger lurking in the dark, and it sends the signal to produce all the chemicals to fight off the attack or run for your life. But the threat doesn't materialize, you don't run or fight burning the adrenaline, so the chemicals stay in your body, and they accumulate, causing stress and anxiety.

Sometimes we don't even know what is causing our stress; a multitude of worries, negative thoughts, and horrible scenarios assail us. Your brain doesn't know the difference between a real threat and your imagination of dire possibilities. It reacts exactly the same. So I have come up with a system to deal with them. When you are filled with anxiety, stress, or worry, my suggestion is to ask yourself these questions:

1. What is the worst that can happen?
2. What I can do about it at this time?
3. What am I actually afraid of?

For instance, suppose you are worried you will lose your job.

What is the worst that can happen?
Your answer could go something like this: "If I lose my job, I will have no money, be unable to pay the mortgage, become homeless, and die of hunger" (translation in your brain: famine is coming—prepare!). Now, determine whether this is actually possible or if your mind is playing tricks on you, frightening you needlessly. It is important to analyze which part of the worry is a possible scenario and which part is just your imagination running wild.

When we are worried, we tend to think of horrible, improbable outcomes and have the emotional reactions as if they were true. For example, when my husband took longer than usual in getting home, I used to go straight to *He has surely crashed and is lying dead somewhere* or *He was kidnapped and is being brutally tortured* instead of the much more plausible *He stayed late at the office* or *There is a lot of traffic.*

Remember that your brain doesn't really know the difference between imagination and reality, so having catastrophic fantasies will trigger negative emotions and drain your energy. It is better to think of more plausible, less tragic alternatives and wait for more information or the real answer instead of tying yourself up in knots for what most often is nothing. When you have a reasonable, plausible scenario, think what you can do at this moment to either prevent the catastrophe or solve it if it happens.

What can I do about it at this time?

In the losing-your-job worry, you can think of proactive steps to take to avoid the worst-case scenario: *I can finish the project my boss asked of me instead of worrying,* or *I will look for alternative job options in case I do get fired.* In some cases, the answer is *I can do nothing.* In the example where I'm worried that my husband is late, I can't really do anything about it. If you can do something about it, do it, but if you can't, there is nothing worth worrying about. Stick to the most reasonable, plausible explanation and focus on something else until you know more. When you figure this out, you can do some soul searching and go to the root of your fear.

What am I really afraid of?

This is a deep question, and if you're like me, you tend to answer it quickly with something obvious. This is because we dislike seeing into our deepest fears. Your fear is probably unfounded if it is not accompanied by a deeply felt, gnawing feeling of foreboding. You know you have it when you come up with a negative belief about life or yourself, and it resonates deep within you. For example, *If I get fired, I will be rejected and unloved*, or in the husband-is-late scenario, *I can't live without him. I will die and cease to exist*. In both cases, you can see that the cause of the fear, and therefore the cause of the stress, is an emotional one that has less to do with getting fired or your husband being in a car crash (which are not very common occurrences), and more to do with fear of rejection and loss.

For emotional triggers, taking a step back does wonders. I got very angry with my spouse one time when he confirmed our assistance at a party without consulting me first, and I wasn't feeling up to it. I could feel myself boiling with rage. (I have an issue with feeling ignored.) Instead of lashing out at my husband, I took a couple of minutes to look deep inside and ask myself what really made me angry. Was it really the party or the fact that I did not feel important or loved? Once I got to the core feeling, I could fill that emotional need for myself. Our core issues are usually love, recognition, belonging, or well-being.

Then, when you have taken care of you, you can channel your anger into something useful, like setting limits *I really don't feel up to going to the party, you go and excuse me please*; or telling your spouse what you really feel and need. For example, you can say, *The fact that you didn't consult me about the party made me feel unloved by you. Please give me a hug and a kiss, and tell me you love me, and next time think about me and ask me*. Normally, the other person will comply happily with your need if it is a direct request spoken sincerely and reasonably, and without criticism.

It is my experience that when you take a step back, go into your awareness, and stop the chaos of the mind for a second, you can really see yourself, your core emotions and fears, and your vulnerability. Facing those with honesty empowers you to respond proactively. As long as you believe that you are the victim, and you stay within the never-ending loop of negative thought patterns and beliefs, your body will comply with your beliefs and give you a terrible time. You need to go deeper within yourself to see your true personality, to determine what really frightens you, and to overcome it. Only then can you stop playing the role of victim. Only then will your body feel better as it complies with new, healthier thought patterns and emotional well-being.

For example, in the scenario where my husband didn't ask me about the party, my mind went off into something like this: *I can't believe he didn't ask me. Of course, he only thinks about himself; he always ignores me. Can't he remember to care that I get sick and can die if I get tired? He doesn't care for me at all!*

What can we see in this inner monologue? First, it is a mental construction. I do not know if any of this is even true. Second, it says more about my own insecurities and fear of being ignored than it does about my husband. Third, I am going into the role of victim, to which I react with anger, which is natural, because feeling like a victim implies there is some outside force attacking me; therefore, I use anger as a defense mechanism. So when I scream at my husband in a rage because he forgot to consult me, I'm not really shouting at him. I am defending myself from a perceived (and probably false) attack.

Being the witness to your own self-awareness helps you recognize this pattern. Only then are you able to work on your insecurities and fears, and use the released energy of the anger to talk calmly to your husband about how his forgetfulness touches you in your weak spots. This immediately takes you out of the victim mindset and makes you the boss of yourself again.

This, however, takes practice. At first, you will go through the whole show before you can get calm enough to take a step back and see what happened. When you get more practice, you can catch yourself sooner and use the emotions released for your benefit instead of letting them get the better of you. Emotions are like the waves in the sea—they come crashing upon you, overtaking you completely, and then they recede. Let them. Emotions are only damaging to you when you try to control them or suppress them. If you are feeling sad, be sad, very excruciatingly sad; cry it out and let it recede. Watch how it is impossible to keep feeling sad if you let it out. You can only keep feeling the emotion when you feed it. Watch how you feed your emotions with your thoughts. When you stop the thought, the feeling will run its course and recede.

Even better, when you identify the negative thought pattern, think positively instead. There is always something good in your life, even if it is small. Think of the good things, make a list of them, and be grateful for them. I love what Carla Ulbrich in the afore mentioned book *How can you Not Laugh at a Time like This*, says about gratitude:

Having a grateful heart turns you from a downward spiral of pain and self-pity into an upward spiral of gratitude and possibility. . . . When you look for what is good, you start noticing more good things, and that gradually changes the habit of complaining to one of celebrating.

CHAPTER 5

Vanquishing Negative Emotions

As we discussed in the previous chapter, emotions are, at the physical level, chemicals produced by our brain in response to stimuli, be it something that is happening outside our body or in our own mind. At the energetic level, emotions are vibrations, frequencies at which you are resonating. It has been amply proven that emotions color our experience of life, thereby defining our reality. If we change our emotional response to a certain situation, we change our experience of that situation, affecting our definition of reality.

When an emotion is expressed in your physical body, you have already experienced it on a mental level. Therefore, the chemicals of that emotion (for example: adrenaline for fear and cortisol for stress) are running through your bloodstream. You have to let the emotion run its course and fade along with the chemicals. Since emotional responses are so critical to our well-being, we must learn to manage our emotions at the physical and the mental level.

The Physical and Mental Level of Emotions

When you are feeling a strong emotion, you are reacting to something. First, determine whether the trigger of that emotion is happening in the outside world or in your mind. For example, if you come very close to being in a car crash, this is happening in the real world, and the surge of adrenaline prepares you to react to the situation. This is a response to an outside stimulus. If you are lying in bed remembering a past car crash you were in and worrying that it might happen again, that is not really happening; it is in your mind, and the resulting adrenaline when you picture the crash is wasted energy. Your reaction to situations occurring in the outside world usually cannot be controlled or altered, as they are part of your innate life-response kit. You have to let those emotional reactions run their course, not feeding them with thoughts, just expressing them in a way that doesn't hurt or scare anyone.

However, the things that are happening in your mind can be changed. Emotions that result from thought patterns are made by habit. You actually have connections in your neurons that favor some emotions and not others, called neuronal pathways. That is why people can be described as angry, sensitive, sad, happy, and fearful. These neuronal pathways are the most usual response you tend to have toward life events. Habitual thinking makes stronger pathways, so for negative responses, we have to break the negative patterns and establish new positive pathways in our brains. New habits will strengthen the new positive pathways, and disuse will weaken the old negative pathways. This will encourage healthier emotional responses, which will make your experience of life better.

Emotional responses create patterns of behavior, which in turn makes whatever you are feeling "true" in the real world. For example, if you have a constant stimulus, like pain, to which you react with fear, every time you feel pain, your brain will produce the adrenaline and cortisol chemicals, and you will be truly afraid. Constant fear results in hopelessness and a feeling of helplessness in life as a general outlook.

If you can change that response from fear to assertiveness, chances are you will be much more able to deal with your pain, making it a completely different experience for you. You will remember the emotion associated with the occurrence, and that will define you in life, not the actual circumstance. In the first reaction, you experience yourself as fearful and life as hopeless, but in the second reaction, you experience yourself as assertive and life as a learning experience that makes you strong. The actual pain in both reactions is exactly the same. What would you rather think and feel about yourself and life?

To illustrate this, remember in the part about my story when I managed to put my feet down on the floor and felt a horrible pain like pins and needles? My reaction to this pain was, the first day, helplessness. I cried out and waited for someone to help me back up, unable to do anything for myself. The next day, when I felt anger and used that emotion proactively, I could feel the pain and stay with it, managing to stand up. It hurt with the same intensity both times, but my experience of this pain was completely different.

Since emotions are automatic responses triggered from deep beliefs, we have to change this process so that it occurs in the conscious mind, not the subconscious mind. This process is a reflexive reaction anchored in the beliefs we made about the world during our childhood experiences.

Therefore, the first step in changing our emotions is recognizing them. After recognizing them, we have to determine the belief that is triggering the emotion. Then we have to decide if what we believe is true.

Let's look at this process using the example from the previous chapter of being angry with my husband:

I am angry because I believe he doesn't consider the limitations of my condition when he is making plans.

In my unconscious mind I have a belief that I am invisible and unloved and he triggers these beliefs and the emotional response to them when he does this.

Is this true? Am I invisible? Am I really unloved? No.

Therefore, my angry reaction is unwarranted. Nothing has meaning in and of itself. We attribute meaning to situations and circumstances. In this light, we can see how we construct our own reality through our belief system, the one we created in early childhood.

Childhood experiences = beliefs = thought patterns = emotions = behavior = how we perceive our experiences = how we color our reality.

Let's consider an example of how this self-fulfilling prophecy works:

When I was three years old, I had an abusive teacher who shouted at me every time I spoke up or complained, which made me feel misunderstood and alone. I started to believe that speaking my mind and complaining was wrong, and I was bad for doing it. I thought of a better strategy of staying quiet, and it worked; she stopped shouting at me, making this behavior efficient, so today, as an adult, I dare not complain or speak up, because I feel guilty and bad if I do. The bear-it-quietly behavior yielded better results in the past, so I stick to it. My experience of the world is that it is better to keep things to myself, so I do not speak up, and this makes me feel misunderstood and alone. This brings us full circle, making my reality what I already believed it would be, which further strengthens my belief that this is the way things truly are. No one will ever understand me or be with me if I speak up and complain.

Positive emotions make us feel good because they produce the beneficial chemicals of serotonin and endorphins in our brains. We want more of these emotions. Negative emotions are thus named because they make us feel bad; they deplete our energy and produce chemicals designed to fight our way out of a threatening situation or flee it. These chemicals, if not used in fighting or running, remain in your system and can be draining. We want as little of these emotions as possible in our lives.

Unexpressed emotions become stuck energy within our bodies. This energy is recognized by your immune system as "the enemy," but you can't attack negative energy with immune blood cells, so the excessive production of these cells circulating in your body in response to this stuck energy needs to find a target. This is what those cells are designed for. So they search, find, and attack whatever comes across their path.

Unfortunately, they can't attack the person or situation that made you feel the negative emotion, neither can they attack the negative emotion itself, so they go for a kidney or whatever other organ, instead. The body perceives the stimulus, and your brain identifies it, classifies it, and translates it into an emotional response. When you have the emotion, there are three possible outcomes:

1. You stay quiet and do not express it = stuck energy = illness.
2. You express it physically = crying, shouting, or being aggressive. Usually results in fights and unsatisfactory relationships, which leads to new negative feelings.
3. You identify the emotion, do something to restore your inner calm, and express it verbally without the drama. This is obviously the best option. You can't do this in the moment you are feeling the emotion. You should retire from the situation, identify the emotion, do one of the following options to calm down, and process the stuck energy. Determine what you want to say to the other person—what made you angry, hurt, or upset— then talk about it calmly.

Identify Negative Emotions

Okay, so how do we change our negative emotions? First, we identify them. Here is a list of human emotions and a brief description of them:

- Abandonment: feeling alone and uncared for
- Unrequited love: lack of love and caring
- Anxiety: state of agitation, fright, and restlessness
- Apathy: lack of interest
- Arrogance: feeling superior to others
- Yearning: desperate desire to get or achieve something
- Disgust: repugnance toward something
- Jealousy: envy of another; suspicion that our loved one is with someone else
- Conflict: internal contradicting forces that cause anxiety
- Anguish: acute distress, suffering, or pain
- Confusion: lack of clarity, doubts
- Guilt: feeling responsible for a fault
- Dependency: needing the protection or help of someone else
- Disconsolate: lack of comfort by another
- Despair: losing hope; feeling helpless
- Unprotection: not feeling protected and secure
- Contempt: lack of appreciation
- Deception: lies, infidelity, not being honest or truthful
- Stress: demanding more of yourself than you are capable of doing
- Lack of control: feeling a victim by circumstance

- Victim: feeling attacked by a person or circumstance and being unable to resist or defend yourself
- Failure: lack of success, frustration, and the certainty of a negative outcome
- Humiliation: motive that damages dignity and pride
- Helplessness: unable to do something about your situation
- Indecision: doubting what you should do; unable to make decisions or take responsibility
- Dissatisfaction: lack of satisfaction, feeling something should be different from what it is
- Insecurity: lack of security and protection
- Anger: lashing out; defensive, violent reaction
- Lust: excessive desire of something
- Fear: alertness and anguish over a threat, real or imagined
- Nervousness: agitation, nervous excitement
- Obstinacy: extreme perseverance, to the point of foolishness
- Hatred: intense and uncontrollable feeling of rejection and aversion
- Pride: arrogance, excessive self-esteem
- Loss: deprivation or lack of something you had previously
- Worry: being fearful of some possible future outcome or unknown event
- Rejection: lack of acceptance or admission; resistance to something that is present
- Suffering: pain (can be physical or emotional)

- Sadness: affliction, anguish
- Shame: a feeling brought on by committing a fault or a dishonorable action (shyness can be the outward manifestation of shame)
- Envy: wanting to have something or be like someone else
- Loneliness: feeling like no one understands you and you are alone, even if surrounded by people
- Hopelessness: lack of hope; seeing the future as dire
- Frustration: wanting something and being unable to achieve or have it
- Resentment: past anger that doesn't dissipate or resolve
- Panic: acute fear
- Phobia: irrational fear that is always present

To Release:

The first step is to recognize what you are feeling, remember, no feeling is good or bad, it just is.

Then identify what circumstance brought up this feeling for you.

The third step is to identify the belief behind the emotion:

I feel_____.

The reason I feel this way is because_____.

This means _____ to me.

After identifying the negative belief about yourself, ask the following questions:

Is this real, or is it only in my mind?

If it's real, can I do something about it?

Most of the time it is not real; it is a belief based on early negative experiences. If it is real, address the person or situation provoking the emotion. If it is something you can control, figure out what to do and then do it. If it's something you cannot control, accept it and move around it.

For example, suppose I go to the doctor and he is not listening to me; he dismisses my symptoms as unimportant or nonexistent. He keeps his eyes on his computer and just says an occasional "ah." This makes me angry because it makes me feel unimportant. I use my formula:

Is this real?

Yes! This situation is real, and I can address it directly: "Doctor, I feel very angry right now because it seems as if you are not listening to me, and that makes me feel unimportant."

A real situation I cannot control, but I can manage: I feel frustrated with my knees because they hurt and I can't get things done. This means to me that I'm useless. Is this belief real? Yes, in part. It is true that my knees hurt too much to get things done. It is not true that I am useless. Can I do something about it? No. Not right now. So I have to work around it. What can I do instead? What can I do that will be easier on my knees today? Maybe I have socks to darn or emails that need answering.

A situation that is uncontrollable and inevitable: I am in the middle of the supermarket and my knees are in agony, but I can't sit down, and I must buy groceries today. I can ask for a wheelchair or scooter, ask for help, take a painkiller, or buy only the essentials to hurry up the process.

When you are in a similar situation, promise yourself a treat when the ordeal is over. Treat yourself kindly, and try to avoid the frustration; it will definitely not help at all! Think of positive things that will happen when you manage this task, and congratulate yourself for every step. Lower your expectations to the minimum; make tiny goals, take baby steps, and be very forgiving and loving with yourself. Then, when the situation has been dealt with, you can do something about the belief that you are useless. You can recount how you dealt with it and see that although your performance was not optimal, you could still do something. You are not useless; you just were not at your best today. This is updating the belief.

Change the Beliefs That Feed Your Thoughts

If you find that your emotion is being fueled by a negative belief, you have to change it, update it. First, come up with a positive belief and a positive emotion that you want instead of the old negative ones. If my belief is "I am a bad person for complaining, and others will shout at me when I do. I feel alone and misunderstood," I could choose something like "I can speak up, and people will listen and love me regardless of my complaints. I feel that I belong now, and others understand me."

The following are various methods to change these beliefs. Use your felt sense or your intuition to choose the best one for you. If you haven't discovered your felt sense, you can try each of these until one works for you, or just go for the one that sounds best or easiest at this time.

Negative emotions are erased by gratitude.

When you feel depressed, angry, or sad, take a moment to pause and reflect. Think of one or two things that you are grateful for in your life right now. One of them can be just to be alive, no matter the circumstance. Another example can be something beautiful in your life, like someone who cares about you, or a beautiful sunset or flowering plant in your backyard. It doesn't have to be earth shattering or transcendental. Think your grateful thoughts and then close your eyes and say them mentally, slowly, being aware of your body, and feel the gratitude in your heart. Let the feeling of gratitude spread to every organ and every cell of your body. Give yourself at least thirty seconds to feel grateful for each thing on your list. When you feel you have let the gratitude spread, open your eyes and observe the change. If you are not yet spontaneously smiling, think of one more thing and do the exercise again. Observe the change in your mood and in your outlook on life. You can do this short, helpful exercise many times throughout the day.

When you feel hopeless and useless, send gratitude to your body.
At those times when you feel ill and things ache and are uncomfortable, take a minute to be grateful for what doesn't hurt. Take inventory of your body. You are probably very aware of what is painful or uncomfortable. Let those body parts recede in your consciousness. Pay attention to the parts that are not painful and are working as they should. Focus on them completely. Do this with at least three parts or organs of your body, and thank them for doing their job

well. Remember, cells are living beings, and they are all doing their best for you. We never pay attention to what is working properly, and we never take into account that when one organ or member is weak, the rest of the body is working overtime to support life. Be grateful to them for that. Acknowledge them for it.

Next, focus on your whole body. Visualize it as a team in which the stronger members help out the weaker ones. Observe how the whole team is doing what it can to be there for you; acknowledge and be grateful for it. You can do this exercise with your eyes open or closed, and even in the middle of an activity when the aches are especially bothersome.

Send gratitude to your immune system: a fun imagination exercise.
The immune system is the armed forces division in your body. You have thought of it as an enemy living inside you, but actually, it is not trying to hurt you; it just got confused as to which parts it encounters are part of you and which aren't. Think of your flare-ups as episodes of friendly fire. One of your generals is absent-minded and gets confused easily. Remember, your thought patterns trigger emotions, which trigger chemical outpourings in your body, which can further confuse this absent-minded general of yours and send him into war mode. He is over reactive and hypersensitive. Maybe he is in the wrong career; he should have been an artist with that sensitivity! But he chose the military and is in charge, but you are the commander in chief of your armed forces, and it is your job to ease your general and make him stand down from all out war to a relaxed peace time mode.

How will you do this? Not by talking to him aggressively or being violent! You have tried that. Being angry at your own immune system doesn't do anything to help matters. Let's try a different approach:

Visualize that you are in the Oval Office sitting behind your desk. You call in the rogue general who has declared war on one of your states. You can imagine that state as a large one or a small one, according to what is being triggered in your body. Say the joints are the Hawaiian Islands, and the general has deployed all his forces to the islands and directed them to attack. You have to convince your general that the islands are not the enemy; they are peaceful islands full of palm trees and coconuts, and surrounded by lovely beaches with friendly people relaxing on them.

Talk to your general; befriend him. Thank him for trying to protect the country. Remind him that his heart is in the right place, but he got the target wrong. Imagine going up to him and patting him in the back for being willing to risk his soldiers' lives in your defense. Then tell him that Hawaii is not the enemy; in fact, the entire country is at peace. There is no enemy, no war, and he can stand down and let the troops have a piña colada and lay on the beach now. They have done their duty and they deserve a break. Visualize your oversensitive hyper-reactive general and his reaction to your friendly words. Watch how he relaxes and smiles as all the stress drains from his war mode stance.

You can have fun with this exercise. Tell him some jokes; take him to lunch. If you have an active imagination, you can even visit Hawaii with him: look around, visualize the beaches and the sunshine, and enjoy the sun and waves with your general.

Think of different places for different body parts. Be creative. Remember, you are working with the right side of your brain, and this is where the imagination and symbolic thinking live. The right brain does not understand language or orders; it speaks and understands symbols and attitudes, and it responds to suggestion in the form of images. The more vividly you engage in this imagination exercise, the better your right brain will receive the message and act on your instructions, calming your immune system in the process.

Let go of worrying about things you cannot control.
Place your thumbs inside your ears on the ear basin (not in the ear canal), and place the rest of your fingers behind your ears. Rotate your fingers gently in a circular motion. As you visualize your worries, one by one, think about the following:

- What you CAN do about this
- What you are willing to do at this moment and what can wait
- Choose ONE action for each worry or thing that you CAN COMFORTABLY DO. Visualize yourself doing it and see how doing this makes you feel, if bad, choose another action, if good, proceed. When you open your eyes, write these positive actions on your to-do list in the order of importance or timing (what is more urgent in time and what can wait).

Let go of fear.

There are many fears, and it is important to identify what your core fear is in any given situation. Most of our reactions are fear based, but we seldom admit to being fearful. Everyone is afraid, and fear is very important in our basic biological set of emotions. Thanks to our fears, we are cautious, we take care of ourselves, and we try to avoid painful experiences. We are even conscious of others out of fear—fear that we won't be accepted or loved, fear that we will be rejected or attacked. We fear pain, we fear death, we fear all that we cannot control, which is almost everything in life. Fear takes us away from danger, or it tries to. That is its function. Fear becomes a problem when we fear things that exist only in our minds, and when we make up stories that keep us awake at night, dreading the future. That is when fear is not useful to us; it becomes a hindrance, an obstacle to overcome.

To conquer our fears, first we have to identify them. Here is a list of the most common fears:

- Abandonment
- Death/loss
- Sickness
- Pain (physical, emotional, or mental)
- Violence/aggression/war
- Old age/impotence
- The unknown
- Success/failure
- Abundance/poverty
- Being loved/not being loved

- Being yourself/rejection
- Loving
- Commitment
- Men (father)
- Women (mother)
- Being dependent/independent
- Sex/sexuality
- The future
- Responsibility
- Power
- Money
- Chaos
- Heights/falling
- Open spaces
- Closed cramped spaces
- Animals
- Driving
- Flying
- Punishment/hell/guilt
- Natural disasters
- End of times/apocalypse/ Armageddon
- Supernatural phenomena (aliens, ghosts, witchcraft, bad luck)
- Supreme being
- Criticism
- Losing control
- Being dirty/contaminated
- The dark
- Fire

- Water
- Being alone
- Change
- Abuse

This list is by no means exhaustive. There are fears of almost everything under the sun! Even the sun itself! Find yours if it isn't on this list. Once you identify what you are truly afraid of, that which is sustaining your negative beliefs and behaviors, you can transmute your fears. Transmutation is the power of change. Remember, energy cannot be created or destroyed; it can only be transformed. In this visualization, we are transforming the energy wasted on your fear and investing it in something positive that you want, such as feeling better or diminishing a specific pain, or a goal you wish to attain:

Visualize your fear as a symbol; it can be a color, an image, a sensation, or a word.

Close your eyes and make yourself comfortable. Concentrate on your breath as you breathe in and out calmly and deeply. Visualize the symbol of your fear in clear detail. Visualize a purple flame in front of you, the flame of transmutation. This purple flame has the power to change things into that which you desire. Visualize the symbol of your fear going into the flame, and watch closely as it changes. It is becoming something different, using that same energy to create something new and exciting, something you desire.

Watch as it transmutes and when, like a butterfly after its metamorphosis, it exits the cocoon of the purple flame, it is renovated, changed, brilliant, and new. What comes out of the flame represents that which you want. It can be a color, an image, a sensation, or a word. Now it is positive, something you truly want. Visualize as this new symbol, in all its brilliance, enters your body again, filling you with positive energy, the sensations associated with that which you want. How do you feel now that you have that which you desire? Let yourself feel it in all of your body clearly, deeply.

When you have the clear feeling all over your body, open your eyes. Look at the situation that caused you fear, and notice the changes in how you think about it, how you feel about it now.

Do the Mayan Breath Exercise to set intentions.
This exercise gives power to your intentions:

1. Think of something you want right now, and think of an image that represents it. For example, my intention could be "I want to have more energy," and the image is me jumping up and down.

2. Take your dominant hand (if you are right-handed or left-handed) and do a "taking in" motion as if you were pulling the energy of the universe into your mouth as you breathe in through your mouth. Imagine this breath going up to your mind and setting your intention (the image that represents what you want in this moment). Exhale through your mouth as you move your hand outward giving your intention back to the universe.

Now forget about your intention, knowing it is in good hands, and go on with whatever you were doing.

Practice this fast dissolution and integration exercise.
This exercise is taken from *A Course of Happiness* by Ricardo Eiriz, but I have modified it slightly. For this one you will need a magnet no greater than 1000 gauss with clear south and north poles.

1. Identify the negative emotion you are experiencing and its founding belief (the first exercise).
2. Pass the north pole of the magnet toward you, from the center of your forehead between your eyes up and over to the back of your head, and as far down your spine as you can go while saying, "I am free of the emotion of____ and the belief that _____". Do this ten times.
3. When you finish, say out loud, "This emotion and its belief have been liberated."
4. Integrate the new belief with positive emotion: Now think of something positive that counteracts the negative emotion. Put all your fingers together, tips touching, about one inch from your temples. Repeat the positive belief statement until you actually believe it; you will feel different when you do. When you feel convinced that you believe the positive phrase, bring your fingertips to rest on your temples and let yourself feel the positive feeling associated with the new positive belief you have integrated. Feel it in all of your body,

and enjoy this positive feeling for a moment and then open your eyes, taking your hands away slowly.

5. Take a moment to feel the difference in your emotional state before and after this exercise.

Keep a gratitude notebook.

When you have a negative belief and you feel its corresponding emotion, think of at least three things that you are grateful for in relation to this situation. For example, suppose you have this thought: *I am frustrated with my knees because they are painful, and I can't get things done.* Think of things related to your knees that you are thankful for. It could go something like this:

1. I have had worse pain than this, and I am grateful it is not that bad.
2. I have legs to walk on.
3. I was born in the era of the painkiller, and I can always take one if it gets too bad.
4. There are people willing to help if I ask them to.
5. If I can't complete the errand of buying groceries, I can ask for takeout or ask my neighbor to share her dinner.
6. I am grateful to be alive and able to make it this far.

Think of as many as you can. If you have time, write them down. I find it helpful to always keep a gratitude notebook with me so that I can jot them down to read again later. Let yourself feel the gratitude of these things. When you feel grateful, you cannot feel any negative emotions, because gratitude dissipates them.

Choose Happiness

Yes, happiness is a choice! We make the choice to be happy each day of our lives. When faced with any circumstance, you can pause and choose to be happy again, step by step, moment by moment. When you do this with awareness, you change your energy vibration from whatever you are feeling to being happy. It takes strength to choose happiness when you don't feel well, but it is possible. Your attitude determines your happiness. The attitude has to be that everything happens for a reason. Everything is for your higher good, and there is a gift in every situation; you just have to find it. Ask yourself:

1. What is good about this situation? What is the gift?
2. What is not good about this situation?
3. What can I do to make things the way I want them to be, having fun while I'm doing it?

It takes willpower to choose happiness. You have to take responsibility for your own happiness. We are all ultimately responsible for our own lives and the way we live them. This exercise just takes that responsibility into account and shows you that you have a choice—you always have a choice as to how you will respond to the circumstances surrounding you. Rose Kennedy said something along the lines of "it doesn't matter what happens to you; what does matter is how you react to what happens to you." She didn't have an easy life either, so if she could believe that, so can we. This is choosing how you react to your life and circumstances. Choose to be happy.

Liberate Negative Emotions

This exercise is based on Chloe Wordsworth's Resonance Repatterning method and modified to do it on your own at home. When you are having a very strong negative emotion, take a pause and follow these steps:

1. Feel where the sensation is in your body. You might feel a knot in your throat or a hole in your chest. Think of the possible meaning of where and what you feel associated with the emotion.

2. Put your hand or hands on the area where you feel this emotion in your body.

3. Use your breath to exhale the negative emotion and inhale its opposite. You can think of a color associated with the emotion and visualize it leaving your body every time you exhale. Think of a healing color and breathe that in to fill the empty space left by the color of the exhaled negative emotion. Breathe in the healing color and breathe out the color of the negative emotion. Continue until you have completely replaced the negative color with the healing color.

4. When this is complete, close your eyes and let your body move of its own free will. The movement has to come from inside you. Don't force it; let it happen of its own accord. It can be small or big, it can be silent or accompanied by sound, anything that you feel like doing, do it.

5. When the movement stops of it's own accord, think of the need behind the emotion. What did you need that

you didn't get? Visualize an image that symbolizes this need and integrate it into the part of your body where you first felt the negative emotion.

Example:

I feel terribly angry with my child because he is refusing to walk, asking me to carry him, and I am exhausted.

1. I feel the anger in my jaw when it tightens.
2. I put my hands on either side of my jaw.
3. I imagine the color red for the anger leaving as I exhale and the color green coming into my jaw when I inhale.
4. When my jaw is suffused with green, I move my body as it naturally wants to; maybe I shake my arms and legs and moan out loud.
5. I needed understanding and compassion instead of demands. For me, compassion is symbolized by an open hand. I visualize the open hand going to my jawline.

Take a moment to see if you feel different now toward your child. You will probably find that you can talk to him/her calmly and express your feelings and ask for his/her cooperation.

Orient your body and your life.

Feeling sick and overwhelmed can make us disoriented in life. When we are disoriented, we experience negative emotions such as confusion, lack of focus, forgetfulness, and frustration. When this happens, we need to pause to reorient ourselves.

When we are oriented toward life, we naturally see and act toward that which nourishes others and ourselves. We feel oriented toward that which gives us purpose in life. The following exercise is taken from *Quantum Change Made Easy* by Chloe Wordsworth, and is slightly modified. It is very easy to reorient yourself when you feel lost; just pause and do the following exercise:

1. Sit down comfortably and close your eyes.
2. Breathe slowly and rhythmically through your nose. When you inhale, expand the ribs and abdomen; when you exhale, contract the ribs and abdomen.
3. Every time you exhale, relax your body from your head to your toes; relax your face, eyes, jaw; relax your chest, upper back, shoulders, and neck; relax your lower back, abdomen, and hips; let go of the tension in your thighs and lower legs. Feel your feet firmly planted on the ground, connecting you to the earth, sustaining you.
4. Focusing on your heart, inhale love and exhale love, making your heart center grow with every inhalation until you encompass yourself, the place you are in, and the people who are there with you. You can continue until you encompass the whole world if you like.
5. Feel yourself 100 percent present in your body, emotions, mind, and soul.
6. Open your eyes and look at your surroundings with relaxed eyes, taking in the beauty of what you see. Recognize how it feels to be oriented.

CHAPTER 6

Staying Well, Living Life

It is essential on the path to recovery to see that hope exists and that choice is real, even if small. Getting these two concepts in your head and the convictions in your body are the first steps to living how you want to live and doing what you want to do. Let's start with the most obvious and bothersome symptoms so you can reestablish yourself as the driver in your own system.

In this section, I will discuss the most common symptoms of lupus and explain what has worked for me to relieve them. If I get more than two symptoms or one of the dangerous ones, such as pain in the heart, kidneys, or lungs, I visit the doctor. Natural remedies are good for daily preventive care, but doctor-prescribed medication can save your life in a crisis. I use cortisone only when I get symptoms, but that is just my crazy approach. My doctor knows this, and even if he doesn't agree with me, he can see that I am living normally, holding it together as it were, so he sort of lets me do my thing now. He still supervises me, and if I don't feel well, I go to him immediately. Talk to your doctor and come to an agreement with him/her to lower your medications little by little while you try alternative means of keeping your body in balance and well-being.

Tips for Minimizing Physical Symptoms

Skin Breakouts: Bathe less frequently and oil your body

Water and soap have harsh chemicals, and when your skin is acting up, they will make it worse. Space your baths to every third day at the most, use fragrance free baby wipes for the parts you do need to clean, and oil your skin. For me, cold pressed extra virgin olive oil works best, but it does make me smell like a salad, so you can also go for coconut or grape seed oil. Almond oil is also really good but a little thick; try them all and use whatever works best for you. You can also add a few drops of scented essential oil, such as lavender, to your moisturizing oil. Another tip is to pour the contents of a vitamin E capsule directly on your damaged skin, which helps it to regenerate faster.

A very good way to avoid soaps and chemicals is to bathe with oatmeal. If you like baths, there are oatmeal preparations ready to use in pharmacies (like Aveeno oatmeal bath). If you shower you can use a handful of raw oatmeal in a soft cloth as soap. When wet, it will release a milky substance that alleviates rashes and itchiness. Cornstarch used as powder also helps, especially in areas that tend to sweat, like the armpits, the inner thigh, the feet, and everywhere you have a rash.

Keep your skin covered when you are out, as the sun is an irritant and trigger for lupus. Try to avoid chemicals on your skin, including those found in sunblock, moisturizers, makeup, soaps, and deodorants. Use all natural products instead. When you have to use cleaners and detergents, wear cleaning gloves. It works best for me to put on thin cotton gloves, and over those, I pull on rubber cleaning gloves.

Be aware of the clothes you wear, as natural fabrics like cotton and silk are less irritating and softer on the skin. Try to avoid synthetic fibers, especially if they itch. Wash your clothes with natural detergents. Try to avoid using bleach and fabric softeners.

Mouth and nose sores

These are telltale signs of an acidic system. Try the alkaline diet described in the next section of this chapter, and brush your teeth with baking soda instead of toothpaste. It is less aggravating and it helps to balance your pH. The drugs prescribed for lupus tend to acidify the system, so you need to help yourself with diet. Calcium supplements (and even antacids such as TUMS) also make the system alkaline. If you have sores inside your nose, keep it well moisturized with the oil you use, which helps the mucus membrane recuperate faster.

Colds, viruses, and respiratory infections

As a preventive measure against bacteria and viruses, use colloidal silver, one drop in every nostril and about ten in the mouth every night. Colloidal silver is a natural antibiotic that will clear out any viruses you may have acquired during the day. Don't overdo it though, as it is a heavy metal. Echinacea drops or supplements and good old-fashioned vitamin C are always good boosts. However, vitamin C causes your system to be more acidic; therefore, if you have nose and mouth sores, do not take vitamin C.

Keeping your throat warm is always a good way to alleviate sore throats. I'm a great lover of pashminas and scarves, even in the summer. Air conditioning makes for harsh temperature changes when you come in from the outside. Always carry something with you and wrap it artfully round your neck in air-conditioned or cold environments.

Viruses enter the body through the mucus membranes in the nose and mouth, and they usually lodge in the nose and throat where they reproduce in your own cells. Keeping your mucus membranes clean and moisturized is a good repellent of viruses. Any enclosed space with lots of people and strong air conditioning is a prime flu contagion space: airplanes, crowded bars, restaurants, churches, your workplace, especially if it is filled with people in cubicles in one big room. Wash out your nose and moisturize it at least once a day and remember to use your colloidal silver drops, which work wonders for prevention. These will keep most viruses from reproducing inside you.

Someone in my support group for lupus shared that tea made with fresh ginger root with a bit of lemon and natural honey helps decongest the chest. Cinnamon tea made with a cinnamon stick, honey, and lemon is very good. For throat pain, make a mixture of equal parts apple cider vinegar and natural honey, and take little sips of this all day. Honey is a natural antibiotic, so it figures prominently in all respiratory infection remedies.

Essential oils, like eucalyptus, rosemary, and mint help open stuffy noses. Rubbed Mentholatum (like good old-fashioned Vicks VapoRub) on the throat and chest help with congestion. There is also a Mexican traditional remedy in which you boil a pot of water, drop in eucalyptus leaves, rosemary and mint (and even a dash of vodka), get a towel to cover your head and the pot, and inhale the vapors (don't burn yourself, wait until the temperature is tolerable) and let all the mucus blockage just drip out of your nose into the pot. Do not go out in the cold after doing this; go right to bed! And please dispose of the contents of the pot.

Joint pain

Cold and hot compresses help relieve joint pain. I have also found rubbing them with menthol or essential oils (Just's Oleo 31 works really well) to be effective.

Keeping your joints warm is always better than keeping them cold, so if it is cold outside remember to cover your knees or any joint that tends to be bothersome. Yoga, tai chi, and qigong move all the joints, which helps to keep them flexible. (I have provided an explanation of these in the next section of this chapter.) If you are too exhausted to do any of these, just do gentle rotating movements of all the joints in your body to the extent you can.

I take glucosamine and chondroitin supplements every day because they help the cartilage regenerate after a flare-up.

Linseeds are reputed to help with strengthening cartilage, and they are also a good source of natural fiber.

Herbal remedies work well for the joints, specifically Arnica, because it combats inflammation. You can take it in a homeopathic form or apply it topically in extracts, oils, or poultices. You could also get the dried plant and make an infusion of it.

Bruises

Spontaneous bruises are common and usually not dangerous unless you get a blood clot from them. If there is any pain close to the bruise, go to the doctor. If not, it will probably fade on its own. Arnica is also good for bruises, as are warm baths, for they relax the veins and make circulation easier, which helps the bruise fade faster.

Migraine

I recommend taking a painkiller immediately, before your headache gets bad. Migraines are caused by the swelling of a nerve in your head, mostly by the auriculotemporal nerve. It runs over your ears, down the jawline, and back to the base of the head. Massaging it in a downward spiraling motion will help with the swelling. It is easy to find; feel for the painful cord on the sides of your skull. Also, massage your temples in a gentle circular motion.

Sometimes migraines are caused by overcharging the large intestine meridian (Chinese medicine). Press the point where the thumb and index finger bones meet. If that area is painful, give it a firm massage until it releases the tension. You can also look for other points on this meridian and find the one that's painful (look for the meridian charts on line, I included a link in the Resource section); the OUCH point is the one that needs help! Give it a massage, adjusting your pressure from light to medium or firm depending on what is right for you. I have provided more information on acupressure in the next section of this chapter.

Kidney problems and urinary infections

Take natural diuretics every day to help your kidneys get rid of extra fluid. Black tea, coffee, and pineapple/parsley smoothies are all natural diuretic drinks, so if you are partial to any of these, go ahead. Also hibiscus tea or water is a great diuretic. For urinary infections cranberry juice can be a good aid. A traditional Mexican remedy is making tea out of corn silk to cleanse the kidneys.

Sometimes urinary, vaginal and some respiratory infections are a byproduct of yeast infections (candida albicans). Test yourself for this fungus by spitting into a quarter of a glass of water and seeing if your spit floats on the surface (good), or if it develops root-like strings or sinks to the bottom of the glass. The glass has to be clear so you can watch what is happening from the side. If the saliva drops, follow the candida diet for one to three months until your spit stays floating on top of the water. This diet will allow your intestinal flora to flourish while inhibiting the growth of the candida albicans. Remember that sugar causes candida to reproduce, and most processed foods have added sugar. The candida diet cuts sugar intake to a minimum, including starchy vegetables and fruits.

For an excellent guide, the one I follow when I have a candida infection, I suggest www.thecandidadiet.com. You can use this site or ask your doctor for the diet.

Hair loss

If I had a cure for this, I would be a millionaire! However, it is one thing to have alopecia, which is the condition of becoming bald by complexion or genetic baldness, and another to lose your hair because of lupus. The latter hair loss is reversible, for you don't have alopecia; you have lost your hair because the skin on your scalp is acting up, because of the medicines prescribed to you or because your energy is low and the body shuts down all systems that are not needed to sustain life (growing hair is not necessary for life). Look at your scalp. If it is red, swollen, has a rash or sores, and your hair falls out because of this condition, you will have to heal the skin on your scalp before your hair will grow back. All the skin remedies I have mentioned are effective on the scalp too.

If your hair is falling out in bunches, ask your doctor if it's a side effect of any medications you are currently on. Prednisone makes your hair fall out, but when you lower your dosage, the hair will grow back. If it isn't a rash or the medications, then you are very weak right now, and you need to get your general energy levels back up. Rest a lot, and do all the sequences of the twenty-six Jin Shin Jyutsu energy locks every day. (These are explained in the next section.) Collagen supplements will help to regenerate the hair when your system is ready for it. Meanwhile, you can experiment with different looks: wear turbans, bandanas, wigs or hats, you can cut your hair short to relieve weight, or if the case is extreme, even shave your head completely as some celebrities do.

Insomnia

It doesn't seem fair that when I most need rest, it is very difficult to sleep, and insomnia can be extremely frustrating and stressful. For me, anything is better than not sleeping. I try the natural remedies first:

- Lettuce infusion
- Valerian extract (tincture or herbal caplets)
- Melatonin dietary supplements
- Relaxation techniques

If these do not work, I go for the over-the-counter sleep aids, and if my insomnia is chronic and ongoing, I ask my physician for a prescription medication. Exhaustion is one of the main triggers of lupus, so rest is crucial for your well-being. Make sure you get at least eight hours of sleep.

Progressive relaxation technique:

Lie down in your bed, ready for sleep. Close your eyes and concentrate on your feet. Tense them, opening all your toes, and flexing your foot. Keep your feet tense for two breaths, and on the third breath, exhale as you relax them completely. Next, focus on your lower legs: tense them, and on the third breath exhale, relax them completely. Then focus on your thighs: tighten your thigh muscles, tighter, tighter, and on the third breath exhale, let go of them completely. Then tense your buttocks and relax. Next, focus on your belly: tense all the muscles in your belly, even your rib cage, and relax. Then, focus on your back; tense the muscles and relax. Focus your attention on your shoulders and arms. Shrug your shoulders, making tight fists, and on the third breath exhale, relax completely, making them completely comfortable. Then go up your neck, tense all your muscles, even raise your head, and on the third breath exhale, relax your neck completely. Now focus on your face: make a pout with your mouth, scrunch your eyebrows and close your eyes tightly, tenser, tenser, and relax completely.

Check your body again in a sweeping manner, from your toes to your head, adjusting any part that is not completely comfortable, letting go of any residual tension, and then focus on your breath, breathing slowly and deeply, but effortlessly. Then focus on your mind, on your thoughts. Imagine that your thoughts are clouds; you are gazing up at the sky, watching as the cloud-thoughts drift by without you engaging them. Just watch them float in, pass through your mind, and float out. Keep doing this until you fall asleep.

Fever

If your fever is high and medication is not working, take off all of your clothes and soak in a lukewarm bath with a bag of ice on your head, even if you are shivering. My nanny used to warm my feet, saying that would draw the fever down to the feet. For this remedy, lie in bed lightly dressed, uncovered, and put on really warm socks and maybe an electric cushion or blanket on your feet. Place an ice bag on your head. This does seem to work a little. The idea here is to cool your head since high fever is dangerous to the brain. The idea behind warming your feet is that, apparently, the body has a hard time keeping your head and your feet hot at the same time, so if you heat your feet, your head will have to cool. If your feet are also burning up with fever, this remedy will not work. Let me caution you against submerging your body in a tub of ice: even though I was given this treatment as an infant, and it probably saved my life, I think this is only a last resort, for it can seriously shock the system. The decision to use this treatment should only be made by a doctor and medical staff in a hospital setting.

Photophobia (sun sensitivity)

Unfortunately, for photophobia, the only option is staying out of the sun or covering up completely if you need to go out. Remember that photophobia changes, depending on your general well-being. Try, every day, sticking your hand out of a door or window, wherever it will be in full sunlight, to determine how strong the sun is that day, and take the necessary precautions depending on your daily tolerance. You can always do the general well-being techniques every day until you get stronger and better.

Anemia

Besides taking vitamin and iron supplements, a diet rich in red meat and dark green leafy vegetables will keep the iron in your blood at normal levels. You should always eat a healthy diet as a general rule, but especially at those times when you are anemic; make sure everything that goes into your mouth is restorative to health. Your body needs to be well nourished to function, and it is already compromised with a confused immune system. Help it to help itself. Be conscious of what you put into your body. Remember that it has to process all foods, and this takes energy, energy you can't waste on processing junk food. Unless the craving for a certain junk food is truly strong, it isn't worth the energy it takes to process it. If the craving is too strong, go ahead and indulge a little because abstinence produces stress, and stress is worse for lupus than junk food.

Alternative Treatments, Therapies, and Diets

Chronic illness is usually dealt with in psychotherapy by improving the quality of life within the possibilities and constraints of the patient's condition. The diagnosis of a chronic illness can cause panic, feeling you have been given a death sentence. But it can also create relief, because the patient can now explain his/her symptoms by assigning a label to them and know that those symptoms are real.

In many cases of chronic illness, especially in so-called "Invisible Chronic Illnesses," or ICIs, the symptoms appear and disappear, and the disease is not visible or predictable, nor is it localized. This is the case with lupus. So many times, the sufferer doubts whether his/her symptoms are real. It is easy to doubt your mental sanity when no diagnosis is forthcoming. Then, the diagnosis causes depression, anguish, and hopelessness because now the patient knows the symptoms are real and incurable. She will then have to cope with those symptoms, on and off, for the rest of her life.

It is very important, from a mental health standpoint, to put these feelings into words and concepts so that you can work with them. We have to remember that any illness, especially if it is chronic, affects the whole system—the patient, the family, and the social group. Ideally, every member of the support system will work through the feelings brought about by the disease.

Unfortunately, psychological help is not readily available. Most times the specialist, when finally found, has to deal with physical and emotional symptoms, and they are usually not equipped to do both. Patients, their families, and their social group are left to fend for themselves with all the emotional overcharge the diagnosis brings. They also have to deal with the ongoing symptoms and the frustration of the unending cycle of invisible illness—flare-ups and remission. If you don't get professional psychological help, you can use any of the techniques in the preceding chapter to start dealing with all the negative emotions caused by your diagnosis.

Having gone through this myself, and still dealing with the aftermath of my original diagnosis and ongoing symptoms, I have tried every available treatment and alternative therapy out there, both for emotional distress and for physical symptoms.

As you have probably gathered by now, this condition has made me a spiritual seeker, as well as a healer, and my own guinea pig in trying out alternative approaches. As I said at the beginning, I have tried everything possible to keep myself healthy and well. Mine is an extensive but not an exhaustive list. I would be the last person to discourage exploration, but do be careful with yourselves, as not every alternative therapy is a good one for you. It seems that in this day and age, new healing practices and methods are launched and sworn by every day. Most of them are based on ancestral knowledge but are slightly modified, renamed, and launched as a new method, or based on modern technologies that attempt to use these wonderful advancements for health options. Most of the modern technological healing techniques are unproven, but as we have seen with technology in other areas, I believe they have great potential.

Ancient practices are still alive because they work. They are based on ancestral knowledge passed down from one generation to the next, so they tend to be effective, but of course no treatment is infallible. Because this is uncharted territory, I advise anyone who is willing to try new treatments to use her intuition or felt sense to navigate these very ample and sometimes confusing waters. I have tested all the practices I recommend in this section and have felt improvement on some level within my body. Every person is different, however, and you might have different results. Please use your own intuition and/or felt sense to choose those that are useful to you, being very attentive to how they make you feel. They should always be for the better, never for the worse, and you are the best radar for that which is beneficial for you.

The following is a synopsis of the various treatments that are most effective and beneficial, for me, at relieving symptoms of lupus.

Resonance Repatterning. Resonance Repatterning integrates an understanding of psychology, the ayurvedic healing of ancient India, the Five Element system of Acupuncture and modern research on the brain and vision (along with Energizing Options using light/color, sound, movement, breath and energetic contacts) to create extraordinary change in people's lives. Chloe Faith Wordsworth, the founder of this system says that all change depends on changing what we resonate with -- that our resonance with unconscious negative beliefs and feelings underlie every problem we have. When we change this unconsious resonance, we change our lives.

NAET. Dr. Devi Nambudripad's discovery, which she named Nambudripad's Allergy Elimination Techniques (NAET®), is an innovative and completely natural method for regaining better health and effectively relieving allergies.

It is an allergy treatment method based on the diagnosis of allergens by applied kinesiology followed by treatment consisting of energy techniques, diet and acupressure to remove the patient's sensitivity to the allergens. I have had it done, and I would advise it. It is always better to have the fewest irritants possible in your immune system! I had a lot of allergies removed by this method, and my overall well-being definitely increased.

Manual Lymphatic Drainage (MLD). Created in 1932 in France by Emil and Estrid Vodder. MLD is a type of gentle massage intended to encourage the natural drainage of the lymph, which is an integral part of the immune system. Manual lymph drainage uses a specific amount of pressure (less than nine ounces per square inch) and rhythmic circular movements to stimulate lymph flow.

Lupus tends to cause the lymph system to clog up, which causes painful swelling. Everything you can do to alleviate swelling will have definite positive effects. This gentle massage is not painful, even if you are very sensitive to touch, and it helps with the correct functioning and flow of the lymphatic system.

I have an MLD massage every week, and when I'm not home and can't do them, I definitely miss them terribly.

Biomagnetism. The official website, Biomagnetism USA, defines it thus:

> *Biomagnetic Pair Therapy or Biomagnetism is a therapeutic system developed by Dr. Isaac Goiz Duran, MD based on his discovery of the first Biomagnetic Pair (BMP) in 1988. It's the use of magnets, of a minimum of 1000 gauss, placed by pairs in specific areas of the body to fight viruses, bacteria, parasites, and fungus, which are the main causes of most illnesses. Dr. Isaac Goiz Duran MD has also discovered BMPs for glandular dysfunctions and other imbalances not caused directly by pathogens.* (http://www.biomagnetismusa.com/)

If you can have a biomagnetism practitioner work on you, that is highly recommendable, for there are many pathogens that do not give any symptoms, but they do activate the immune system, and as we all know, this is never good for a lupus patient. If you can't have a session by a professional biomagnetism practitioner, I have come up with a placing of magnets that will help with your general wellbeing.

To practice biomagnetism on your body, you will need four magnets, preferably healing grade magnets (1000 gauss) that clearly distinguish between north and south poles. This placement of the magnets is of my own device and it works for almost any condition, even when you're feeling tired, overcharged, and overwhelmed. Place a south magnet on each sole of your feet, a north on your belly button, and the last north on the crown of your head. The direction I mention is the one touching you, so for the soles of your feet, have the south poles on your skin; for your belly button and the crown of the head, have the north poles facing you.

Leave them on for twenty minutes and then remove them. Be careful not to place the magnets near any electronic device, because the magnets will cause those to malfunction. Do not leave them on your body for more than twenty minutes, and do not experiment on yourself by putting the magnets anywhere else on your body. You can get the magnets at www. ResonanceRepatterning.net/estore or at any place that sells biomagnetism magnets. If you can't find any of these, you can even get magnets at hardware stores. Just make sure the north and south poles are clearly marked, and do not use magnets over 1000 gauss!

Reiki. The International Center for Reiki Training defines it like this:

> *Reiki is a Japanese technique for stress reduction and relaxation that also promotes healing. It is administered by laying on hands and is based on the idea that an unseen "life force energy" flows through us and is what causes us to be alive. If one's "life force energy" is low, then we are more likely to get sick or feel stress, and if it is high, we are more capable of being happy and healthy. (http://www. reiki.org/)*

Reiki is defined as energy healing and I find that it makes the body heal faster and gives you a boost of energy when you are really tired. Although having a therapist administer Reiki treatments is preferable, I recommend getting initiated at least to the first level so you can have this wonderful tool at hand (literally).

Jin Shin Jyutsu. The Jin Shin Jyutsu Physio-Philosophy is an ancient Japanese art of harmonizing life energy in the body. Our bodies have energy pathways that feed life into every cell. When one or more of the paths become blocked, the resulting stagnation of energy can disrupt local areas in the body and eventually disharmonize the whole path of the energy flow. Jin Shin Jyutsu uses twenty-six bilateral safety energy locks along these energy pathways. Holding these energy locks with a contact with your fingers brings balance to the mind and body.

It is a very effective energy balancing system, but practitioners are hard to come by. You can do all these energy locks as one of your restful activities to promote well-being. You can also read what they are about and find the one you need according to the symptom you feel if you are short on time.

Detoxification by heat. I have tried temazcal, sweat lodge, steam room, and sauna. Sweating is good to get toxins out, so doing any of these periodically is helpful. Just be careful not to overdo it and to keep hydrated. They are especially useful when you cannot exercise or when you have no other detoxifying methods available.

Urine-based vaccines. No information is available online for this therapy. I used it as an experimental treatment, and

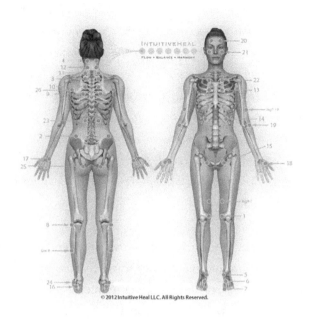

Jin Shin Jyutsu chart of 26 energy locks and functions
(taken from the Ituitive Heal web page).

apparently it wasn't very successful. The inflamed skin on my hand did abate, but I'm not very sure it was due to the vaccines. Besides, I have not heard about this therapy since then, so my advice is to skip this one.

Acupuncture. The following description is taken from the MNT Knowledge Center page:

Acupuncture involves the insertion of very thin needles through the patient's skin at specific points on the body — the needles are inserted to various depths. We are not sure how acupuncture works scientifically. However, we do know that it does have some therapeutic benefits, including pain relief and alleviation from nausea caused by chemotherapy. According to traditional Chinese medical theory, acupuncture points are located on meridians through which qi vital energy runs. There is no histological, anatomical or scientific proof that these meridians or acupuncture points exist. Acupuncture remains controversial among Western medical doctors and scientists.

I have found that acupuncture is an incredible healing technique, and I found relief from some symptoms when they were not acute. I use it more as a maintenance method when I feel good or when symptoms are in the early stages. The only problem is finding a good acupuncturist in your area.

Fortunately, acupressure also works, and you can do it on yourself. It works by applying pressure to the meridian points, and it is very helpful when you can identify your particular points (they are usually recurrent). For me, a particularly useful one is the point between the thumb and index finger, which correlates with the large intestine meridian. Pressing and gently rubbing this area in a circular motion is especially good for alleviating headaches. You can find meridian point charts easily on line. Usually the OUCH point is the one you need. Press on the points on the chart for a damaged organ. The one that hurts is your OUCH point, and it needs attention. You can press it or massage it gently, whatever you can take, until the pain starts to subside.

Homeopathy is a form of alternative medicine created in 1796 by Samuel Hahnemann based on his doctrine that like cures like (similia similibus curentur), which means a substance that causes the symptoms of a disease in a healthy person will cure similar symptoms in a sick person.

It has been called a pseudo-science, and there is no scientific proof that it actually works. However, I have felt the beneficial effects, and it does seem to speed up recovery. I have found it useful in managing flare-up symptoms, like skin rashes. The only problem is you have to be really consistent in taking the globules for it to be effective. I would definitely recommend trying it if you can adhere to a schedule and not miss a dose, especially if you have a certain proclivity for symptoms such as swelling of the joints or skin rashes. These symptoms do seem to diminish when you start the remedy as soon as the symptoms appear. Consult with your physician first, homeopathic remedies can interact negatively with medications.

Bach's Flowers. Developed by Edward Bach, an English homeopath, in the 1930s, Bach flower remedies are solutions of brandy and water, with the water containing extreme dilutions of the flower parts. Bach believed that the dew found on flower petals retained the healing properties of the plant. The remedies are intended primarily for emotional and spiritual conditions.

The same applies to this treatment as with homeopathy: you have to be consistent in your use of Bach's flowers, but I have seen great results in my patients emotional reactions when using this therapy, so I recommend it for people who are disciplined in following a treatment regimen.

Yoga. I love yoga! It is the only exercise that does not drain me of energy. I can accomplish other tasks during the day after a yoga session. It keeps my muscles flexible and strong without too much exertion, and all that twisting makes me move all the joints of my body, which keeps them from stiffening. I have tried three variants of yoga, and they are all good. Hatha is slower and less demanding physically, Kundalini deals more with the raising of energy levels, and Ashtanga is more physically demanding, faster than Hatha, and more strengthening than Kundalini. But any form of yoga is great; try them out, or go for what is offered near you. You can also find DVDs and online videos with yoga practices that you can do at home (I offer one in the Resource page).

All forms of yoga are extremely good for keeping the body flexible, which helps to reduce the minor aches and pains of lupus flare-ups. If you try Bikram yoga, practiced at a temperature of 40 degrees Celsius, which is the same as 104 degrees Fahrenheit (very hot), just be careful not to overextend yourself, as it may be more painful than helpful if you do. If your body temperature gets overheated, your immune system could go into defense mode.

Yoga is also practiced as a moving meditation. Since you are moving every part of your body, you can use it as a mindfulness technique and a daily self-assessment to see how well you are feeling that day. Note whether anything hurts, if some part is stiff, or if you feel tired. Yoga will help you monitor yourself closely if you do it with awareness.

Tai Chi. Tai chi is a great exercise because even though you move all your body parts, it doesn't exhaust you since it is done so slowly. It forces your mind into a slower pace, giving you the opportunity to become aware of your body, which helps you monitor it. It is practiced in many parks in the United States; find out if there is a group near you that practices daily. The whole Chinese nation does these exercises every day, so if there is a Chinese community near you, it is very probable they have a tai chi group you could join.

Qigong. Qigong is a type of spiritual practice intended to align the body, breath, and mind for health, meditation, and martial arts training. With roots in Chinese medicine, philosophy, and martial arts, qigong is traditionally viewed as a practice to cultivate and balance qi (chi) or what has been termed as life energy.

Qigong is a great option for exercising while balancing your energy; it is meditation in motion. I had to stop doing it, regretfully, because my knees hurt too much, but I want to try it again now that I am better at not overdoing things. If you have access to any of these practices (yoga, tai chi, and qigong), please try them out. Find the one you enjoy the most.

Ionic Detox. This is a detoxification process by which an ionater machine is placed in a basin of saltwater in which you immerse your feet for thirty minutes. It removes toxins from your body as the ionater releases ions into the water, the polarity is reversed periodically, creating positive and negative ions, which are then taken into your body through your pores. Supposedly, your cells are energized by the ions in the water, which encourages your cells to release oil, acid, fat, heavy metals, and other debris and waste that have accumulated in your cells and bloodstream. The toxins are carried out of your feet and into the water, turning it a bright rust color or a murky brown.

It was impressive to see the water after the detox, and each time I have had it done, the water has never been the same color or intensity of murkiness, but I didn't feel any immediate effects on my well-being. This is another of those harmless treatments you should try if you are curious, but I can't really tell you that it helps.

Traditional herbal medicines. I tried Chinese, Mexican, Ayurvedic, and herbal combinations prescribed by an iridologist and a shaman. These remedies are natural alternatives to medication. After all, medicines originally come from plants, and most active ingredients in medications are found in nature. You have to have a good herb specialist to get what you really need. I do not interchange doctor-prescribed medications for herbal tinctures and combinations. I am not a herbologist, and I do not know any I would trust my life to. However, there are many herbal medicines that are great for alleviating symptoms.

For example, for me, a combination of corn silk and willow bark tea worked well for minor pain and cleansing the kidneys after taking cortisone and other medications. Also, pineapple and parsley water work wonders as a natural diuretic, helping with the swelling produced by the cortisone. Always ask your doctor for any possible interactions between plants and medications before trying any herbal treatment, because they do have active ingredients.

Dietary supplements. I had every recommendation from everyone trying to help, and I swallowed all of them. They only work if you need them; if you don't, you are only overcharging your system, for it has to metabolize all those substances and eliminate them. I would suggest trying them one by one and being very perceptive to how they make you feel. If good, then go on; if bad, give them up immediately. It is always good to check with your doctor before taking dietary supplements because they can interact with medication, sometimes in negative ways.

Diets

They say you are what you eat. I like to think your body can do more with better building blocks. Eating a healthy diet is recommended for everyone. Here again, healthy is personal. What may work for someone won't necessarily work for you. Try different options to see how you do. I have tried the following:

Ayurveda. This is an ancient Indian healing system, based on diet, dietary and herbal supplements, and your personality. Deepak Chopra is a proponent of this method. Wikipedia gives the following explanation:

> *Ayurveda names three elemental substances, the doshas (called Vata, Pitta and Kapha), and states that a balance of the doshas results in health, while imbalance results in disease. One Ayurvedic view is that the doshas are balanced when they are equal to each other, while another view is that each human possesses a unique combination of the doshas, which define this person's temperament and characteristics. In either case, it says that each person should modulate their behavior or environment to increase or decrease the doshas and maintain their natural state. (https://en.wikipedia.org/wiki/Ayurveda)*

The knowledge that Ayurveda gave me about my body type and the foods that are better for me was beneficial to improving my health. Feeding your body foods that are more compatible with it makes it not have to work as hard. Therefore, your body conserves valuable energy that otherwise would be wasted in the digestion and metabolizing of foods that probably are not good for you anyway. However, the particular diet they gave me didn't work for me; it made me feel weak because it was vegetarian. Apart from the results I got, the philosophy behind it makes complete sense to me. I am now very aware of the foods I eat and how I feel after eating them. For me, animal protein and fat are easily digestible and give me energy, whereas too many carbohydrates make me lethargic and overweight.

All-organic diet: I'm sure it is better for you, and if you have the availability and budget, go for it! The fewer toxins you put into your body, the better. I am, however, not a rabid believer anymore. It proved very stressful to adhere passionately to a diet of organic food because it is not available everywhere, and stress is a primary instigator of lupus flare-ups, so that wasn't a good trade-off. Whenever possible, though, I purchase organic foods; when eating out or traveling, I don't concern myself about it.

Candida diet. There is an easy test to know if you have candida: Spit into a glass of water. If your spit floats on the surface of the water, you are fine; if it develops root-like stings or sinks to the bottom, you have candida. Cortisone and other medicines usually prescribed for lupus tend to cause a candida overgrowth in the body because they kill the beneficial intestinal flora, which allows the candida fungus to reproduce without impediment. If you test positive with the spit test, consult your doctor for a blood test. After getting rid of the candida, follow the diet anyway so that it won't come back. A good remedy to keep your beneficial flora healthy is to drink three spoonfuls of fresh, raw potato juice on an empty stomach in the morning. The high glucose level of the potato feeds the friendly bacteria in your intestine; do this after completing the diet. Look for it online at thecandidadiet.com/.

Alkaline (all white) diet. This is not an official diet. I amalgamated it through trial and error. Later I found out that a new tendency in alternative medicine is to say that disease is the effect of acidity in the body. A similar diet is recommended to make your system alkaline again. When I have mouth or stomach ulcers, alkaline foods are the only foods I am able to eat. Alkaline foods tend to be white or pale in color. My guideline is very simple: white foods have no irritants, whereas the brighter the color, the more irritating the food will be to my body. Using this logic, stick to white meats such as fish and chicken, white or pale vegetables (potatoes, corn, zucchini), and pale fruits (apples and bananas).

Most processed foods have chemicals in them that make the body acidic. You want to maintain your body's alkalinity to keep it healthy; therefore, it's best to eat natural foods.

Most fruit is very acid; the milder ones, such as bananas and apples, won't cause pain, and melon can also be good, but pineapple, strawberries, and all citrus foods can be very painful. Try to avoid tomatoes and peppers.

Of course, you will be the judge; if it hurts, stop eating it. Eating acidic foods when you have ulcers aggravates the condition. It can aggravate to the point of having bleeding ulcers that can become infected, which can be very painful.

Be very aware of the effect that different foods have on your body at different times. Remember, your body has different symptoms depending on what it is experiencing at certain times, so what is fine one day may not be good the next. My body tells me immediately if a particular food is not good for me. It has been difficult to get past the "waste is bad" idea, and I still sometimes go ahead and eat it, usually with painful results. Here again, be the judge of your daily tolerance for various foods; be respectful of what your body tells you. When my mouth has ulcers or is very sensitive, I brush my teeth with baking soda because it is not as harsh as toothpaste, and it helps prevent infections in the gums.

Balancing Your Body's Chakras

Chakras are energetic centers within the body. They have been part of the Hindu tradition for thousands of years, and this system has recently been adopted in the West.

Although their existence and importance is not scientifically proven, I have found that keeping these centers balanced and adequately open is a very good maintenance technique. Besides, the practices recommended to balance them and keep them in good shape are not difficult or unpleasant, so please include them in your stay-well routine!

There are seven major chakras in the body: earth, water, fire, air, ether, third eye, and crown. We will examine these in detail and see how each chakra pertains to maintaining a healthy body. This information was mostly taken from a

Resonance Repatterning seminar by Chloe Wordsworth called Transforming Chakra Patterns. But information on the Chakras is readily available and you can also read more online about this method at the official website Resonace Reppaterning.com/.

Earth Chakra

Located at the base of the spine underneath the tailbone, the earth chakra has to do with the function of bodily elimination. Its related sense is smell. The negative feelings that correlate to this chakra are fear and greed. The positive feeling is satisfaction. Its color is red, and its Ayurvedic sound is YAM. Its taste is sweet. It relates to the little finger and your little toe. The earth chakra deals with survival and belonging to a tribe or group, so any threats to your life and a sense of being alone or not belonging affect this chakra.

In my experience, lupus has a direct correlation with the earth chakra because this health condition is always threatening survival. It is interesting that the immune system also pertains to the earth chakra, and is usually hyper-activated, especially in lupus flare-ups. This puts the system at risk. We sometimes tend to feel rejected, attacked, not normal, and therefore, our sense of belonging to our family or group feels threatened. If you don't do anything for any other chakra, you should definitely take care of this one every day!

To balance the earth chakra, do the following:
1. *Polarity touch*: hold your little finger
2. *Food*: sweet foods (rice, dates); foods that grow under the earth (root vegetables, beets, carrots, potatoes); red fruits and vegetables (tomatoes, apples, red berries)

3. *Actions*: walk barefoot on the earth to ground your body or do gardening
4. *Visual*: look at earth and rocks, crystals, minerals, and beautiful landscapes
5. *Dietary supplements*: minerals and calcium
6. *Music*: listen to or dance to drum music (African tribal is great), or anything with a steady beat (move with bended knees and an upward/downward motion)
7. *Movies*: those with a patriotic or family theme (The Patriot, Braveheart).

Water Chakra

Located on the stomach about four fingers below your bellybutton, it deals with procreation and creativity. Its sense is taste. Its negative feelings are cravings and lust, and the positive ones are moderation and continence. Its color is orange; its sound is VAM. It relates to the ring finger and the fourth toe. Salty foods are its jurisdiction.

This center is important to keep balanced if you are doing a creative project or want to get pregnant, as it deals with sex and creativity, as well as sensual pleasure.

1. *To balance the water chakra, do the following:*
2. *Polarity touch*: Hold your fourth finger.
3. *Food*: Water, plenty of it, orange fruits and vegetables (oranges, papaya, melon, peaches, carrots); foods that grow on the earth or close to it (cucumber, pumpkin, watermelon); salty foods and seafood (green algae, fish,

shellfish, miso, soy sauce). Sushi is a tasty option if you feel like you need to balance this chakra.

4. *Actions*: Being close to or in the water; swimming in natural environments is best, such as the ocean or a lake, but a bath also works.

5. *Visual*: Watching the sea, lakes, waterfalls, moonlight reflected in water.

6. *Dietary supplements*: All those made with seaweeds; sea salt.

7. *Music*: Listen to or dance to flowing cheerful rhythms, sensuous music such as rumba, samba, cha-cha-cha, or cabaret. Move your hips in a flowing sexy way.

8. *Movies*: Feminine themes where women discover their sensuality and beauty (Titanic).

Fire Chakra

Located on the solar plexus (where the sternum ends), it takes care of digestion. Its sense is sight; its negative feeling is anger; and the positive ones are forgiveness and tolerance. Its color is yellow, and its sound is RAM. It is correlated with the middle toe and finger (the one you give the finger with!). Its taste is bitter. The fire chakra deals with power and empowerment, with that feeling of "I can." It also deals with fun, parties, friends, recreation, intimate relationships, and interpersonal communication, as well as hugs, friendship, and pleasurable activity.

The fire chakra is usually very low in energy in people with lupus, for it is easy to feel helpless, angry, and unable to deal with life. After the earth chakra, this is the most important to keep balanced so that you always feel like there is something you can do for yourself.

To balance the fire chakra, do the following:
1. *Polarity touch*: Hold your middle finger
2. *Food*: Fruits and vegetables that are yellow (pineapple, guava, pumpkin, bananas); bitter foods, (arugula, spinach, coffee); all cooked foods (meats, cooked vegetables, hot dishes). Hot foods such as peppers, chilis, and hot spices, as well as ginseng, ginger, and cinnamon.
3. *Actions*: Have fun with friends, watch a fun movie, do something you enjoy. Enjoy the sunshine, children playing, talking with friends, and laughing.
4. *Visual*: Light a fireplace, have candles in the room, watch a friendly fire (a campfire).
5. *Dietary supplements*: Ginger, pepper, chili, anything that heats the body.
6. *Music*: Listen or dance to happy, cheerful tunes (like the aptly named "'Cause I'm Happy"). Dance with rapid, jumping-like motions. It's party time!
7. *Movies*: Fun movies or those that imply men finding the true use of power; hero type films; action/adventure movies (Superman).

Air Chakra

At the center of the sternum, in line with the heart, is where the air chakra resides, on the thymus gland. This is also known as the heart chakra. It regulates breathing, the respiratory system, the heart, and the circulatory system. Both these systems never stop working; they have no rest, so it is vitally important to keep them running smoothly. The air chakra's sense is touch, and its feeling is attachment and healthy detachment. Its color is green (for loving others) and pink (for loving yourself). Its sound is YAM, and it relates to the index finger and the second toe. Your mother told you off with this finger; now you know she was speaking from the heart! Its taste is acid.

The heart chakra relates to having meaning and hope in life, and with being able to love yourself and others. Having what is usually termed an incurable illness diminishes our self-image and self-love; we become bitter and feel that life is unfair. With these thoughts, the heart chakra gets hurt and becomes afraid to love others, love ourselves, and even life itself. Also the thymus gland is associated with the immune system, so if you feel unloved or you don't love life, this can affect the thymus' capability for regulating the immune system.

One of the antidotes to these negative thought and emotional patterns is gratitude. The heart fills with joy when you are thankful for what you do have, instead of bitter for what you don't. The feeling of gratitude even helps you to come to forgiveness, of yourself, others, life, even God. Forgiveness is a gift you give yourself, not others, and it is so powerful when it is sincere and from the heart—the whole universe smiles!

To balance the air chakra, do the following:

1. *Polarity touch*: Hold your index finger.

2. *Food*: Fruits and nuts that grow up high (almonds, nuts, all fruits that grow on trees); acid foods (citrus fruits like lemon, lime, oranges); green fruits and vegetables (pistachios, avocado, lettuce).

3. *Actions*: Read self-help literature (you are doing that right now!), enjoy a loving relationship, say positive affirmations to yourself, pamper yourself. Tap your thymus gland with your index and middle finger in a waltz rythm (1, 2, 3...1, 2, 3).

4. *Visual*: Gaze at mountains and clouds; enjoy being outside on windy days.

5. *Dietary supplements*: Everything that is good for the heart, like omega-3 and omega-6; vitamin C also.

6. *Music*: Listen to or dance to love songs, tender music, soft music. Dance slowly, preferably with someone you love!

7. *Movies*: You guessed it! Romantic and inspirational movies, especially those with a happy ending (You've Got Mail, Love, Actually).

Ether Chakra

Located at the base of the throat, the ether chakra deals with communication, listening, and speaking. It deals with the vibration of sound. Its negative feelings are hopelessness and longing for the divine. Its color is light blue, its sound is JAM, and it relates to the thumb and big toe. It takes care of all the joints in the body. Its taste is metallic.

The ether chakra is the empty space before creation, the place of new beginnings, of infinite possibilities. It is the first of the physical chakras, so it is where the spiritual energy enters the body. It is the space of limitless possibilities and timelessness. We who have lupus tend to close it off, for we don't believe we have infinite possibilities; we believe we are unable to do many things.

As it deals with communication, we tend to shut the ether chakra, for we think that others get tired of hearing us complain about how miserable we feel. So we stop communicating, we stop believing in our possibilities, and life becomes a dreary process; every day is the same.

This chakra, when open, gives us the chance to see different things we can do, different options, and roads to take. When we have faith in ourselves and in God, the Creator, the Source, or whatever you want to call the creative energy behind everything we see and are, life has purpose. Everything happens for a reason, and we are here for a reason, an important one. Spirituality becomes tangible in this chakra.

To balance the ether chakra, do the following:
1. *Polarity touch*: Hold your thumb.
2. *Food*: Organic, pure foods, light and easy to digest; beautifully prepared food, with an esthetic presentation; metallic tastes (oysters, rare red meat).
3. *Actions*: Beautify your home, have invigorating conversations, do a spiritual practice such as prayer, meditation, contemplation, or spiritual reflection; move your joints slowly and harmoniously

> (tai chi or gentle circular movements with focused attention).

4. *Visual*: Watch a cloudless sky, harmonious colors, soft light, a sunset.
5. *Dietary supplements*: None.
6. *Music*: Spiritual, inspirational, classical.
7. *Movies*: Inspirational (Chariots of Fire).

Third Eye Chakra

On your brow, a little above the eyes, right in the middle of your forehead, is where the third eye chakra dwells. This chakra doesn't deal with body parts, senses, or tastes. It deals with vision, imagination, and visualizing goals, especially goals with purpose that are part of your mission in life. Its color is dark blue, and its sound is OM.

> *To balance the third eye chakra, do the following:*

1. Do imagination exercises, guided meditation, and visualization.
2. Set goals in line with your higher purpose, with things having to do with service to others, values, your legacy.

Crown Chakra

Located on the top of your head, about an inch above your cranium, is your crown chakra. This is the first point of contact of the energy of the spirit and the body. It is the spiritual chakra and has the highest vibration. Its color is violet, and its sound is a sharp keening sound. It is where the influx of life energy enters the body, and some say it is where the soul leaves the body when we die. It is beyond all senses and emotions. It is peace, devotion, unconditional love, absolute faith.

To balance the crown chakra, do the following:

1. Have a spiritual path and practice your faith through spiritual contemplation, deep meditation, prayer, and devotion.
2. Listen to spiritual music, such as Gregorian chants, church music, and the Ave Maria.

The chakra localization chart (taken from Wikipedia):

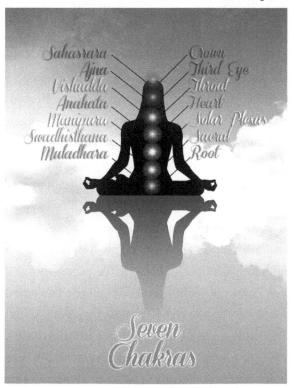

Here is one technique I have found useful to balance all the chakras, but please feel free to explore your own methods if this one doesn't work for you:

Chakra balancing visualization technique

Chakras are energy vortices in certain locations throughout the body. They flow from the center of the body to the sides and from back to front. They each have a color and correlation as shown in the chart and discussed above. To balance the energy of all the chakras, you can do this visualization. You can read it and then do it if you have a good memory, but it is more practical to have someone else read it slowly to you, or record it for yourself.

Get in a comfortable position, sitting down or lying down, with your eyes closed. Relax your muscles and be aware of your breath as you breathe slowly and deeply. Become aware of your body, of your posture; if there is anything tense or uncomfortable, relax or rearrange it until you are fully relaxed and comfortable. Put your attention on every inhalation and every exhalation as it happens naturally, without any effort on your part.

Crown Chakra: Imagine a violet light in the shape and size of a Ping-Pong ball on the top of your head; it doesn't touch your head but floats slightly above it. The crown chakra is where your spirit connects with your body, where you are divinely inspired and have spiritual meaning and purpose. Observe this ball of light and make sure its radiance is strong and clear. If you see, feel, or perceive any cloudiness or weakness, strengthen it with your intention. Make the ball clearer and brighter every time you inhale, and let go of any cloudiness when you exhale. When you feel it is radiant and clear, go on to the next.

Third Eye Chakra: Visualize a channel going down through the center of your body from the crown chakra through the inside of the brain to the spot between your eyes on your forehead. There, imagine a ball of indigo blue light. Indigo blue is the color of the deep sea. Imagine this deep blue ball of light glowing bright and clear in the middle of your forehead. This is your vision center; through it you have vision in life, set goals, and see what lies beyond this moment. If there is anything cloudy or the light is dim, concentrate your breath on it, inhaling brightness and clarity, exhaling cloudiness and dullness, until it is luminous and as clear as the clearest deep ocean, emitting strong light. When this chakra is ready, go down through the channel in the middle of the body to the next.

Throat Chakra: This is a spot right at the base of the neck, where the neck makes that little indentation between your collarbones. Imagine here a light blue ball of light. It is as clear as a summer sky. If you detect any clouds or darkness, exhale them, bringing more clarity and luminosity with very inhalation. This is your communication center; through this chakra you can communicate with others and listen to them, but you can also listen to yourself. When your chakra is glowing with clear light blue energy, move on to the next, down through the channel in the center of your body to the place in the middle of your chest.

Heart Chakra: This chakra is usually larger than the others; it glows green when experiencing love of others and pink when experiencing love of yourself. Focus on the pink aspect, inhaling pink light to the center of the chest, exhaling any emotional pain that may linger there. Spend extra time in this area, giving emphasis to your positive feelings of love for yourself, as well as forgiveness and gratitude. Every time you inhale, bring one of those feelings into your heart center and let it expand throughout your body on every exhalation.

Fill yourself with the energy of the heart, inhaling love and acceptance, exhaling self-pity and judgment, inhaling forgiveness and exhaling control, inhaling gratitude and exhaling recrimination. When your chakra is glowing bright pink and has expanded to the size of your shoulders, and you can feel the love, the forgiveness, and the gratitude throughout your body, move down the central channel into your solar plexus.

Solar Plexus Chakra: This is right below the sternum, where the ribs fan out. It is the mouth of the stomach. Visualize here a Ping-Pong sized ball of yellow energy, clear and strong, like a 100-watt light bulb. Inhale light and energy; exhale darkness and murkiness. Make this chakra strong, and make it emit a lot of light. This is your power chakra; from here, you feel capable of doing things; it gives you strength and power. Inhale yellow light; exhale feelings of impotence. Inhale power; exhale cloudiness and dimness. When it is glowing and you feel stronger, go down through the central line to the next one.

Water Chakra: A little below the belly button (three to four fingers), it glows with orange light. Visualize this orange sphere of light in the center of your body. Clean any dark spots with your breath, bringing in more light, letting go of dimness or dark spots. This is your creative force; through this cha[...] you can manifest and create your own life. Make it bright an[...] beautiful with your breath. When it is ready, go down to the last one.

Earth Chakra: It is at the base of your body, in the pelvic floor, between your anus and vagina. This is your life force, a sphere of light that glows red like the magma of the earth, hot and powerful. Inhale red light and exhale any darkness. Feel the rhythm of the earth in this chakra, the natural cycles, the strength of life that wants to thrive and survive. Embrace this natural force, the will of life to perpetuate itself; make it glow red with that tenacity and strength.

When you are sure it is glowing strongly, take a quick trip back through the central channel looking in on every energy center, making sure they are all perfectly aligned on this central channel, all the same size, like Ping-Pong balls, except the heart, which can be much bigger, and glowing brightly, strongly with no dark sports or cloudiness. When you are back to the crown, breathe differently and open your eyes. Take a moment to notice how refreshed, revived, and changed you feel.

Release negativity and find forgiveness.

You don't have enough energy to hang on to old relationshi[...] regrets, anger, or fear, none of us do. You need all your ene[...] to do what you want in life. The following is an exercise t[...] find extremely helpful, and it is based on the chakras with[...] body. It was given to me by one of my teachers who has [...]en the shamanic path, Leopoldina Rendón, and I have [...]tly modified it.

Close your eyes and visualize a root-like beam of light going from your root chakra to the center of the earth; its color is bright white, quartz like. Make it really deep and strong. Then visualize light energy coming up through the soles of your feet and into your body, traveling all the way to where your belly button resides, making a sort of pool of energy that surrounds you. This energy can be any color you want it to be. It may come spontaneously, or you can choose it based on the chakras and what you feel you need. When you are sitting in a pool of colored light (it has to be clear and sparkling), visualize a beam of golden light coming into your crown chakra through the middle of your body and into the same pool of light, not mixing with the other color, but mingling, like oil and water.

Exhale and send half of the pool of light down through your root into the earth. The rest of the energy will go up to your chakras, starting with the earth chakra up to your water chakra and subsequently higher up. You will "wash" out each chakra with the light you absorbed through your feet, all the way up to your crown chakra. When you get there, let the energy flow out of your crown chakra like a fountain, surrounding your body. Stay there for a few moments; feel your grounding and the protection of the light around you. Outside the colored fountain, imagine an egg-shaped bubble of golden light covering you completely from your feet to your head.

Now, visualize the negative and/or troublesome person sitting on a quartz bench in front of you, also inside a bubble of golden light. Place a cord of rainbow-colored light from your to his/hers. Visualize any emotions related to this person as cars; breathe them out of your bubble and give them back to that person through the rainbow-colored bridge. Leave the colors at the edge of his/her bubble. Then visualize any energy this person may have that is yours; gather it up from his/her bubble and bring it back to you through the rainbow bridge, leaving it at the edge of your bubble for it to take its own place. When you have returned all of this person's energy and retrieved all of yours, say the following in your thoughts:

I am (your complete name), and from whom I am, I decree that I have finished suffering in the relationship with you.

I am me, and from whom I am, I invoke forgiveness for both of us, for all that we have done to each other, and I now leave you in peace.

I am (your name), and I am at peace with you.

CHAPTER 7

Adieu and Godspeed

As I have mentioned before, I have a curious and exploring nature, which has led me into all of these and more ways to keep myself healthy and well. My path of exploration has been complicated and time consuming, so I have tried to make it easier for you. Let this book be your guide to alternative medicine so you can go into this territory with a map of what is out there and what is possible.

I promise you, the reader, that while you try out what I have already tested, I will continue on my quest for optimal health, and I will share all my findings and experiences with you in the future. All the therapies I have mentioned have more formation about them online. I took the most readily available rces to make further research easy and free for you.

134

Don't feel overwhelmed by all the suggestions in this book, they are not intended to intimidate you, but to give you options, for you to find what works for you. An easy way to access all the resources in this book is making a daily wellness routine. The simplest way to do this is choosing one organ or function at a time and keeping to this routine until that organ/function feels better, then chose another one and do a routine for that one. I recommend choosing one physical remedy, one emotional release method, one spiritual practice and one energy technique for each organ/function. You are the judge of what is bothersome to you, and what makes it better, so at the end make an assessment of what worked and what did not. This is an example of a wellness routine, it is best to keep a notebook for your routines, so that you have a reference of how they worked for you for future use:

Wellness Routine: Kidney

Physical Remedy: Drink one pineapple and parsley smoothie for breakfast, hibiscus water in mid morning, and an infusion of corn silk after lunch.

Emotional release: The kidney deals with fear, so ask yourself what is it you are afraid of today. Do the Let Go of Fear section, work through this emotion.

Spiritual Practice: Send gratitude to your kidneys every time you remember throughout the day. Pay special attention to the kidney area in your daily awareness check up, notice any differences in their wellbeing day to day as you follow the routine.

Energy methods: Take special care of your earth chakra (it takes care of elimination), eating foods that activate it, concentrating on actions that strengthen it, like gardening or walking barefoot on grass.

Find the OUCH point on the kidney meridian and give it a short, 2 to 5 minute massage every day.

Daily Stay well routine: Daily awareness check of your body and how it's feeling, with any method you choose (with special attention to the area you are working on). One Jin Shin Jyutsu energy lock (always bilateral), or the 26 if you have time. Food that is good for you. One pleasant activity that you enjoy.

Assessment: Corn silk tea was effective, hibiscus water was too acid and hurt, so I changed the hibiscus water for more corn silk tea. I found many fears and had to work through them all! The chakra balancing work was difficult, because it's winter, so I changed the walking barefoot on grass for buying a quartz crystal and placing it where I see it easily throughout the day. Three points on the kidney meridian were painful, so I massaged them all, one in the morning, one in the afternoon and one at night. Sending gratitude to my kidneys made me more aware of them and this helps in keeping tabs on their wellbeing. I found no time to do a full meditation, so gratitude had to be enough.

———

I hope you find resources that work for you, and I especially hope, with all my heart, that you will find solace, relief, and hope in these pages. I will be writing more techniques and fresh insights on my webpage befriendingthewolf.com and on the Facebook page with the same name. There you can find all my contact information for any questions, suggestions, or just for chatting. I wish you a long, happy, symptom-free journey!

Resources

Bibliography

Cavataio, Neva, *If it Doesn't Go Away, Come Back*, ebook, Copyright 2012

Combs, Pamela Miracle *Battling Lupus, A Survival Guide,* ebook.

Donoghue, Paul J. PH.D, Mary E. Siegel, PH.D., *Sick and Tired of Feeling Sick and Tired, Living with Invisible Chronic Illness*, W.W. Norton & Company, New York – London, copyright 2000, 1992.

Frankl, Viktor, *Man in Search of Meaning, From Death-Camp to Existentialism,* Buccaneer Books, Copyright 1946, 1959, 1962.

Moore, Sharon, *Lupus, Alternatives that Work,* Healing Arts Press, Rochester, Vermont

Ross, Jenny, *The Lupus Answer, A Holistic Lupus Diet & Treatment*, ebook, copyright 2012

Ulbrich, Carla, *How Can You Not Laugh at a Time Like This?*, Tell Me Publishers, New Haven, Connecticut, Copyright 2011.

Wordsworth, Chloe, *Quantum Change Made Easy*, Resonance Publishing 2008, Scottsdale, Arizona, Second Edition 2010.

Wordsworth, Chloe, *Spiral Up*, Resonance Publishing, Scottsdale, Arizona, Seventh Edition, 2014.

Zippieri-Caruana, Marisa, *Lupus, Real Life Patients Talk*, Copyright 2013, Thoughts and Letters Press.

Web pages (recommended)

Acupuncture: www.medicalacupuncture.org/

Ayurveda: The Chopra Center: www.chopra.com/our-services/ayurveda

Bach's Flowers: The Original Bach Flower's Remedies: www.bachflower.com/

Biomagnetism: For Dr. Goiz's official page go to: http://www.biomagnetismusa.com

Chakras: Chakraenergy.com

The Chopra Center: www.chopra.com/ccl/what-is-a-chakra

Homeopathy: Homeopathic Treatment & Homeopathy Medicine: treatment.hpathy.com/ *Remeber homeopathy can have adverse interactions with medication. Ask your doctor before taking any homeopathic remedy

Jin Shin Jyutsu (R): Jin Shin Jyutsu Pyshio Philosophy: https://www.jsjinc.net. For a chart of points google Jin Shin Jyutsu and go to images.

Ionic detox: Alternative Wellness Center: www. alternativewellnesscenter.org/svc-detox.htm

Manual Lymphatic Drainage: Vodder School for Manual Lymphatic Drainage (MLD) vodderschool.com/manual_lymph_drainage_overview

Meditation:

Synchronicity by Master Charles Cannon: https:// **synchronicity**.org/

Meditation music: www.youtube.com/ watch?v=5PIBMLvcAzc https://play.google.com/store/ apps/details?id=net...meditationsounds...

Guided meditation: www.aham.com/

Meridians:

The Chinese Medicine Meridian System: www.acos.org/ articles/the-chinese-medicine-meridian-system/

The Meridian connection/TCM World Foundation: www. tcmworld.org/what-is-tcm/the-meridian-connection

Namumbripad's Allergy Ellimination Techniques (N.A.E.T.): https://www.naet.com/

Qi Gong: National Qi Gong Association: nqa.org/about-nqa/ what-is-qigong/

Tai Chi: Tai Chi Chuan 24 Steps for Beginners: www. youtube.com/watch?v=P5hvODK2zW4

Traditional Chinese Medicine: Taking Charge of your Health & Wellbeing: www.takingcharge.csh.umn.edu/explore.../ traditional-chinese-medicine

Reiki: The International Center for Reiki Training: www.reiki. org/faq/whatisreiki.html

Taking charge of your Health & Wellbeing: www. takingcharge.csh.umn.edu/explore-healing-practices/reiki

Resonance Reppatterning Institute

http://www.resonancereppatterning.net

Yoga: Yoga Poses: https://yoga.com/poses

Aknowledgements

I want to thank my family for their constant love through my illness and for giving me the space and time to write this book.

My parents especially, who have always supported me, helped and held me and my sons together when things got really rough.

To all my friends who have tried to understand me and the unpredictable nature of my condition, who have loved me even when I could not see anyone or participate in their activities.

The doctors that saved my life, and my head doctor who let me experiment on myself without judgement.

Also, I want to thank Chloe Wordsworth, whose teachings have become part of who I am, as all great teachers and teachings should.

I also want to thank Rick Frishman and all the team at Author 101 that introduced me to my editor, Splitseed and my publishers, Morgan James, N.Y., making the experience of writing to publishing a fun and fast process.